For John Mannix, SM
and Charles Abercrombie, MB

Contents

Humanizing
Healthcare
Reforms

GERALD A. ARBUCKLE, PhD

Foreword by Dr Maria Theresa Ho

Jessica Kingsley *Publishers*
London and Philadelphia

Please see page 10 for a full list of copyright acknowledgements.

First published in 2013
by Jessica Kingsley Publishers
116 Pentonville Road
London N1 9JB, UK
and
400 Market Street, Suite 400
Philadelphia, PA 19106, USA

www.jkp.com

Library of Congress Cataloging in Publication Data
Arbuckle, Gerald A.
  Humanizing healthcare reforms / Gerald A. Arbuckle
; foreword by Maria Theresa Ho.
     p. ; cm.
  Includes bibliographical references and index.
  ISBN 978-1-84905-318-1 (alk. paper)
  I. Title.
  [DNLM: 1. Health Care Reform. 2. Cultural Competency.
3. Process Assessment (Health Care) WA
525]

  362.1--dc23

                              2012030833

British Library Cataloguing in Publication Data
A CIP catalogue record for this book is available from the British Library

ISBN 978 1 84905 318 1
eISBN 978 0 85700 658 5

Printed and bound in Great Britain

Foreword

Healthcare reforms and organizational changes have led to turmoil in contemporary healthcare systems worldwide in the past 15 to 20 years. Significant increases in healthcare expenditure have led stakeholders to question the return on substantial investments in health and focused attention on accountability. Changing population demographics and the growing prevalence of chronic diseases have altered models of healthcare delivery with concomitant, and often dramatic, changes in the structure of organizations, whether by consolidation and mergers, or the restructure of different components of a healthcare system. Among the most difficult of a healthcare organization's challenges in the midst of this turmoil is the identification and clear articulation of the values and goals that unite its members and constituent agencies. Without attention to these values and to the processes for developing a shared understanding of them, organizations are unlikely to thrive and remain resilient in the face of chaos and conflict.

During my 10 years working as a clinician in Australian teaching hospitals and subsequent 20 years teaching medical students and training clinicians and managers, I learned that an understanding of professional cultures and the importance of shared values is critical in caring for those we serve. In July 2011, I met Dr Gerald Arbuckle and discovered, to my delight, that we shared a deep concern to preserve and re-emphasize the importance of values such as compassion, solidarity and social justice. This shared concern forms the focus of this book.

Humanizing Healthcare Reforms arose from the series of lectures Dr Arbuckle presented for the annual D'Arcy Memorial Lectures at the University of Oxford in 2011, based on the theme of 'Healthcare in Chaos: Models in Conflict', because of his published concern that human values must be respected in healthcare reforms.

Dr Arbuckle, a graduate in social anthropology from the University of Cambridge, with postgraduate studies at the University of Oxford, is a highly respected and experienced healthcare consultant for organizations in the United States, Canada, Ireland and Australia. It is this combination of a deep understanding of the importance of values in healthcare, scholarly credentials and a highly pragmatic approach to practice that makes his messages to leaders in healthcare organizations so compelling. The material is deliberately presented through the lens of social anthropology, with the aim of bringing values back into the healthcare debate. His writing style is highly accessible and, to those who have the privilege of knowing him, absolutely consistent with his openness to listening to other viewpoints, strong inner convictions and reflective insights. This is evidenced by the care with which he chose, as an anthropologist, to re-emphasize the Good Samaritan story and its values as the historical founding myth of all Western healthcare.

Clinicians, leaders and managers in public and private healthcare organizations worldwide are facing a formidable challenge that is calling into question their sustainability. Leaders are being called on to account for every aspect of expenditure and activity, and expected to deliver value for money. Consequently, the fundamental message of this book, the centrality of the founding values of Western healthcare, is critically relevant, timely and desperately needed.

Dr Maria Theresa Ho, MBBS (Syd), MHP (UNSW), MD (UNSW)
Formerly Associate Professor and Associate Dean (Learning and
Teaching), Head of the Medical Program,
Faculty of Medicine, University of Sydney
Co-author with George R. Palmer of Health Economics:
A Critical and Global Analysis *(Palgrave Macmillan, 2008)*

Acknowledgements

My particular thanks to Jessica Kingsley Publishers and to the editor Lucy Buckroyd for their encouragement in the writing of this book; to the community of Campion Hall, University of Oxford, for providing me with a hospitable research atmosphere to prepare the book; to Ms Margaret Zucker and Dr Tessa Ho for their patient and detailed reading and commenting on the text.

My thanks also to publishers for permission to quote extracts from the following: C. Anderson *et al. Making Mergers Work* (London: The Economist, 2000), page 3; D. Brooks, *The Social Animal* (New York: Random House, 2011), page 149; R. Hadikin and M. O'Driscoll, *The Bullying Culture* (Oxford: Butterworth-Heinemann, 2000), page 75; R. Pool and W. Geissler, *Medical Anthropology* (Maidenhead: McGraw-Hill/Open University Press, 2005), page 1; F.W. McFarlan, 'Working on Nonprofit Boards', *Harvard Business Review 77*, 6 (1999), page 77; E.H. Schein, *Organizational Culture and Leadership* (San Francisco, CA: Jossey-Bass, 1985), pages 314, 316–317; and P. Drucker, *Managing the Non-Profit Organization* (New York: HarperCollins, 1990), page 45.

Introduction

*Increasingly, anthropologists and health professionals work
hand-in-hand in an interdisciplinary effort to alleviate suffering.
(Robert Pool and Wenzel Geissler)[1]*

The purpose of this book is to examine the ever-increasing
organizational and cultural turmoil in healthcare institutions and to
suggest how reforms based on foundational values can be achieved
and maintained. This will be done particularly through the lens of
social anthropology, the academic discipline that specializes in the
study of culture. However, readers are not required to have prior
expertise in social anthropology. Policy-makers and strategists in
healthcare reform, clinical practitioners, managers, those with the
task of professionally training clinicians, and students, will find the
book especially helpful. Indeed, people in all walks of life who must
lead cultural changes in today's turbulent world will benefit from the
book's theoretical and practical reflections.

The turmoil in healthcare is strikingly evident. In fact, all healthcare
systems are at the crossroads. Changing demographics, new, often
strident consumer demands, severe and increasing government
budget limitations, major global and national economic uncertainties,
and rapid technological changes[2] are placing immense pressures on
hospitals, aged care facilities and other providers of both medical
and long-term care services. Structural reform follows reform with
breathtaking speed. In the British National Health Service (NHS)
significant organizational disruptions have occurred almost annually
since the mid-1980s, due to policy decisions emanating from the
Department of Health in London. Revolutionary restructuring for

---

1   Robert Pool and Wenzel Geissler (2005) *Medical Anthropology*. Maidenhead: Open University
     Press, p.1.
2   Thomas H. Lee, a professor of medicine at Harvard Medical School, concludes that the
     delivery of healthcare 'is fragmented and chaotic, principally because of an explosion of
     knowledge and technological advances'. Thomas H. Lee (2010) 'Turning doctors into
     leaders.' *Harvard Business Review 88*, 4, 53.

the NHS in England[3] was proposed, but subsequently significantly modified, in July 2010,[4] and finally legislated by parliament in March 2012.[5] An editorial of *The Times* commenting on this latest proposal correctly declared that: 'The upheaval will be enormous and chaos is inevitable.'[6] This pattern of frequent policy changes resulting in major organizational upheavals has also characterized public healthcare services in other countries such as Australia and New Zealand. A noted US healthcare expert, Henry Aaron, rather bluntly describes the healthcare of the United States as 'an administrative monstrosity, a truly bizarre melange of thousands of payers, with payment systems that differ for no socially beneficial reasons.'[7]

In fact, throughout the Western world the structural and technological changes in healthcare continue to be so hurried, so multifaceted, so bewildering and unpredictable that the resulting organizational cultural instability has been aptly described as 'simply *chaos* or *white water change*.'[8] To add to the chaos, since the mid-1980s, healthcare has become increasingly market led, rather than needs based, even in countries like Britain, Australia and New Zealand that until recent times, had rejected this approach. Universal healthcare was originally built on values such as solidarity, universality, comprehensiveness, equity and social justice.[9] The emphasis is increasingly on values of the marketplace such as choice

3   Economist Julian Le Grand writes that the changes would not have been revolutionary since they were but a logical extension of previous reforms. From a structural perspective he is correct, but the expected cultural upheaval would have been immense. See Julian Le Grand (2011) 'Cameron's NHS reform is no health revolution.' *Financial Times* (19 January). Accessed on 27 June 2011 at www.ft.com.

4   See Department of Health (DoH) (2010) *Equity and Excellence: Liberating the NHS*. London: DoH. This particular restructuring applies only to England, not Scotland, Wales and Northern Ireland. See Stephen Harrison and Ruth McDonald (2008) *The Politics of Healthcare in Britain*. London: Sage Publications, pp.156–161.

5   Prior to its election in 2010, the UK government promised not to change the NHS, assuring people that the status quo was affordable and would be maintained. However, the Health and Social Care Act, introduced in 2012, is the most far-reaching restructuring of the National Health Service in England since its establishment in 1948.

6   Editorial (2011) *The Times* (18 January), 2.

7   Henry J. Aaron, quoted by John Glasser (2011) 'Keep formation in-house.' *Health Progress 92*, 5, 27.

8   See W. Jack Duncan, Peter M. Ginter and Linda E. Swayne (1995) *Strategic Management of Health Care Organizations*, 2nd ed. Oxford: Blackwell, p.9; Thomas H. Lee and James J. Mongan (2009) *Chaos and Organization in Health Care*. Cambridge, MA: Massachusetts Institute of Technology, pp.3–18.

9   See Allyson M. Pollock (2005) *NHS plc. The Privatisation of Our Health Care*. London: Verso, p.83.

and competition, in opposition to the original founding values.[10] Paradoxically, at the same time, concerned reformers in the United States are struggling to modify their long-established, highly expensive model of healthcare that is built on the competitive values of market economics to the detriment of millions of people who cannot afford private insurance. They are not calling for the end of autonomy, diversity, individuality or self-determination in healthcare, but for an increased focus on the values of solidarity and a greater concern for the common good.

Impact on staff members and patients

Given the constant change in healthcare, it is not surprising that staff members can feel overwhelmed and suffer the symptoms of change overload, such as widespread cynicism, absenteeism, bullying and other dysfunctional behaviour (see Chapter 4).[11] Clinicians can feel disempowered, managers can feel harassed by politicians to meet impossible targets. Staff members have been heard to exclaim: 'We've seen it all before, nothing works, just ignore it and keep your head down as it won't last.'[12] Ultimately, this behaviour negatively impacts on the welfare and safety of patients. In Britain, the Department of Health in 2005 considered it necessary to publish a document to remind NHS staff members that their primary focus of concern must be the patient![13] In the United States clinicians have had to be reminded that they must behave, not as hosts of patients and families in the care system, but as 'guests' willing to listen to what people are saying.[14] A report in 2008 into the state of public acute care hospitals

10   See Julia Neuberger (2002) 'The Values Project.' In Bill New and Julia Neuberger (eds) *Hidden Assets: Values and Decision-Making in the NHS*. London: King's Fund. Stefan Collini, University of Oxford, forcefully argues that the British government views even universities as engines of economic growth and technological advance. Traditional non-economic values such as the love of learning are being sidelined; see Stefan Collini (2012) *What Are Universities for?* London: Penguin.

11   See David J. Hunter (2002) 'A Tale of Two Tribes: The Tension between Managerial and Professional Values.' In Bill New and Julia Neuberger (eds) *Hidden Assets: Values and Decision-Making in the NHS*. London: King's Fund, p.62.

12   See Kieran Walshe (2003) 'Foundation hospitals: A new direction for NHS reform?' *Journal of the Royal Society of Medicine 96*, 108.

13   Department of Health (DoH) (2005) *Creating a Patient-Led NHS: Developing the NHS Improvement Plan*. London: DoH.

14   See Donald M. Berwick (2009) 'What "patient-centered" should mean: Confessions of an extremist.' *Health Affairs 28*, 4, 560.

in New South Wales, Australia, concluded that their workplace culture is now 'characterised by lack of respect and trust, absence of empathy and compassion, inability to celebrate the success of others, failure to communicate, and a lack of compassion.'[15] A 'new culture needs to take root,' declared the report, 'which sees the patient's needs as the paramount central concern of the system and not the convenience of the clinicians and administrators.'[16]

Cultural analysis

How is a new culture in healthcare to take root? To answer, we must clarify the meaning of culture and the values that must underpin healthcare reforms. The neglected issue of culture by healthcare planners and practitioners is the major obstacle to organizational change. We ignore culture at our peril. Without an informed understanding of the complexity of culture and the behavioural consequences of cultural change, many avoidable disasters will continue to occur, jeopardizing the safety and welfare of patients. Since the mid-1980s there has been a seismic shift among anthropologists in the understanding of the meaning of culture (see Chapter 1), but much of this rethinking is hidden away in professional journals and books not readily accessible to the non-specialist reader.

The words 'culture' and 'structure' are frequently used interchangeably in contemporary planning reports of healthcare services. This can have unfortunate consequences. Organizational structures are *visible* formal directives covering areas such as who is in charge, how people must act in an organization, the rules governing the handling of technology and so forth. A culture, on the other hand, is far more complex than the popular definition, 'what people do around here'. Rather a culture tells its members how to *view* the world and, above all, how to experience it *emotionally*. In this sense, a culture primarily resides deep in the hearts of people, not in their heads as structures do. It is the emotional glue that binds people together, giving them a comforting sense of meaning and

---

15   Peter Garling (2008a) *Final Report of the Special Commission of Inquiry Acute Care Services in NSW Public Hospitals, Vol. 1, Special Commission of Inquiry.* Sydney: NSW Government, p.416.

16   Ibid, p.3. See also Robert Francis (2010) *Final Report of the Independent Inquiry by the Mid Staffordshire NHS Foundation Trust.* London: Stationery Office.

predictability, often in a confusing and changing world. Cultures cannot and do not change quickly. It is relatively simple to set out administrative directives for organizational or technological changes, but unless the culture of the people involved is addressed, such changes, no matter how logical and reasonable they appear on paper, are bound to be resisted.

The common failure to appreciate the complexity of culture is understandable. We are accustomed to seeing entire landscapes being destroyed and redeveloped over a short time. In our naive understanding of the power of structural and technological change, it can be assumed that the same destruction and redevelopment can take place just as briefly within the organizational cultures of healthcare. It is considered that the symbolic landscapes of peoples can be destroyed, the familiar sights, sounds and routines in which they are nurtured and work can be obliterated overnight by an official administrative decree, without particularly negative consequences. This is not so. Symbols, myths and rituals, which form the heart of a culture, are not replaced as quickly as buildings or landscapes or mass produced as neatly as automobiles, toothbrushes or medical thermometers. The uprooting of the inner framework of a culture destroys people's stable sense of belonging and their individuality. Most are bound to experience periods of intense loss which can lead to all kinds of dysfunctional behaviour. Hence, the urgency for leaders to grasp the meaning and power of culture. Management expert Edgar H. Schein rightly ends his landmark study of leadership and culture with this warning: 'Leadership and culture management are so central to understanding organisations and making them effective that we cannot afford to be complacent about either one.'[17]

Return to founding values

What human values should underpin and guide the reform of healthcare cultures? In the United States the business ethic has come to dominate healthcare and it is in constant danger of becoming the measure of healthcare in other countries of the Western world. The

---

17   Edgar H. Schein (1985) *Organizational Culture and Leadership*. San Francisco, CA: Jossey-Bass, p.327.

United States spends two-and-a-half times as much as its counterparts in Europe. This enormous cost, while millions of Americans have gone without healthcare insurance, is primarily due to the fact that healthcare is mainly in the hands of investors. They view medical care as 'a commodity in trade rather than a right.'[18] People are to be treated as commodities. The same commercialization of healthcare has become an increasingly popular view among politicians and policy makers in England and elsewhere.

Given this growing emphasis on market economics in healthcare, the comments of Michael Sandel,[19] in his 2009 Reith Lectures about the need to develop a new politics of the common good, are particularly relevant. He asserts that 'an era of market triumphalism is at end.' Markets, he says, 'have become detached from fundamental values, that we need to connect markets with values...to shore up values of responsibility and trust, integrity and fair dealing; to appeal, in short, to personal virtues as a remedy to market values run amuck.' He continues, that 'the better kind of politics we need is a politics oriented less to the pursuit of individual self-interest and more to the pursuit of the common good,' and calls for 'a more robust public discourse – one that engages more directly with moral and even spiritual values.'[20] Even at the World Economic Forum held at Davos, Switzerland, in 2012 many conferees openly questioned the values of free market economics. In healthcare, the need to refocus on moral and spiritual ideals means returning to a mission based on founding values such as solidarity, equity, respect and compassion. People have a right to choose their healthcare services, but the choice must not be pursued at the expense of solidarity, that is, the needs of people on the margins of society. Healthcare reforms cannot succeed until we seriously challenge some of the core values of the market

18 Arnold Relman (2010a) 'Health care: The disquieting truth.' *The New York Review* (30 September), 45, and (2010b) *A Second Opinion: Rescuing America's Health Care.* New York: Public Affairs, pp.15–67. See also Laura K. Olson (2010) *The Politics of Medicaid.* New York: Columbia University Press. Americans spent $2.6 trillion on healthcare in 2010, an astonishing 18 per cent of the GDP. See 'Health care in America' (2012) *The Economist* (4 February), 55. By contrast the United Kingdom spends around 8 per cent of its GDP on healthcare, Australia and Canada approximately 10 per cent of their GDP.
19 Michael Sandel is the Professor of Government at Harvard University.
20 Michael Sandel (2009) 'A New Citizenship.' Reith lectures. Accessed 13 June 2012 at www.abc.net.au/rn/bigideas/stories/2009/2609699.htm, pp.1–2.

place: autonomy, individuality, self-determination and diversity (see Chapter 3).[21]

Structure of the book

The first four chapters explain the meaning of culture and its relevance to particular issues in healthcare, while the remaining three focus on what is required to lead cultural change in the turbulence of healthcare.

Chapter 1, 'Power and Complexity of Culture: Healthcare Insights', defines culture and its constituent elements from a social anthropological perspective. It then sets out, in a series of guidelines, the practical implications of this definition, illustrating the material with examples from the field of healthcare. The culture of an acute care hospital is extremely complex, the hospital employing 40 or more different professions, each with its own subculture. The culture of a healthcare system of a country is, of course, even more complex. The British NHS employs more than 1.4 million people; the public health system in New South Wales, Australia, with 250 hospitals, employs 120,000.

The theoretical insights contained in this chapter form the foundation upon which the subsequent chapters draw.

Chapter 2, 'Healthcare Models in Conflict: What about the Patient?', identifies five models of healthcare: the traditional, foundational, biomedical, social and economic rationalist. Each model resolves the fundamental tension in healthcare, namely that between 'the mission' and 'the business', in different ways. The foundational model, with its emphasis on the values of solidarity, equity and social justice, gives primary emphasis to 'the mission' of healing in decision-making. This is in opposition to the economic rationalist type which emphasizes 'the business' side of healthcare with its values of individual choice, efficiency and competition. The foundational model, while not denying the necessity of efficient business management, assumes

---

21 Tony Judt, social critic and historian, has critiqued the decline of moral values in political life, including debates concerning healthcare, in his 2010 book, *Ill Fares the Land*. London: Allen Lane, pp.106–119.

that the primary purpose of healthcare institutions is the safety and welfare of patients. Mission, not markets, is the principal magnet inspiring passion, devotion and hard work from staff and volunteers.

Chapter 3, 'Tribalism between Clinicians[22] and Managers: Risks to Patients', explains the reasons for the tensions between the two subcultures. Members of each subculture are apt to act like 'real' tribes, with their own values, histories, ways of thinking and rules for correct behaviour. Each tribe assumes that its own way of acting is right and that all those 'other people' are wrong, irresponsible or 'just plain inferior'.[23] For the safety and welfare of patients, it is essential that ways be found to build cooperative teamwork across the traditional boundaries of these subcultures.

Chapter 4, 'Bullying in Healthcare Institutions: An Anthropological Perspective', directs readers to identify cultures that encourage the significant problem of bullying in healthcare institutions. For example, hierarchical organizations where resources are limited and political interference is common, such as are traditionally present in healthcare services, readily encourage bullying. Moreover, healthcare institutions are frequently subjected to structural changes that contribute to job insecurity and work-related stress. All this can lead to, or reinforce, existing cultures of bullying. The chapter ends by focusing on ways to develop a culture of justice in which bullying is not tolerated.

Chapter 5, 'Leading Cultural Change in Healthcare', focuses on the two issues of leadership and cultural change. Policy documents frequently refer to the critical importance of leadership in healthcare reform, but what leadership means in the midst of this complexity and turmoil remains undefined. Often it is confused with management. The chapter argues that for the reform of healthcare organizations a *paramodern* type of leadership is required, that is, leaders who are

---

22 The word 'clinicians' can be confusing. For example, it can refer to medical, nursing or allied health personnel. Likewise, the words 'physicians' and 'doctors'. 'Physicians' in Britain refers to a specific subculture within the medical profession, whereas the term equates to 'doctors' in the United States. Also in the United States there are 'family physicians', but in Britain, Australia and New Zealand they are referred to as 'general practitioners'.

23 Edward T. Hall (1986) *Beyond Culture*. New York: Doubleday/Anchor, p.43; see also Peg C. Neuhauser (1988) *Tribal Warfare in Organizations*. New York: Harper Business, pp.3–7.

able to re-articulate and re-own the founding values of healthcare and apply them creatively to contemporary conditions.

Chapter 6, 'Leading Mergers in Healthcare: Cultural Processes', begins with the harsh reality that the majority of mergers in healthcare either fail or never reach their potential. The most common reason for this is the failure to appreciate the inbuilt resistances to change within cultures. The chapter ends with a series of practical guidelines to guide leaders of mergers.

Chapter 7, 'Faith-Based Healthcare: Case Study', first highlights the importance of faith-based healthcare institutions, such as hospitals and aged care facilities, particularly in the United States, Canada and Australia. There is surprisingly little published on the extent, purpose and contribution of these institutions. The chapter summarizes the advantages of these institutions, but then explains why they face significant challenges. Publicly they emphasize 'the mission', not 'the business', as the driving force in all decision-making. However, this emphasis is under threat from two main sources: rising financial costs and the difficulties of finding and training staff who are willing to commit themselves to the vision, mission and values of the organizations. A series of practical guidelines for those in leadership positions completes the text.

I illustrate the text with examples from my research and experience. I have, for the last 25 years, been an applied anthropological consultant on leadership and cultural change to public and non-profit healthcare systems in the United States, Canada and Australia. My experience in working with non-profit healthcare systems is contained in my book *Healthcare Ministry: Refounding the Mission in Tumultuous Times* (2000). For five years I was a director on the national board of the largest Australian non-profit health and aged care system that also manages five public hospitals. In 2009 I was appointed for three years by the Government of New South Wales as a member of the independent panel that was established to oversee the reform of the public hospitals in that state, following the report by Commissioner Garling.[24] I spent much of 2010 at the University

---

24   See Garling 2008a.

of Oxford researching material for this book and preparing for the Martin D'Arcy Memorial Lectures, presented at the University in Hilary Term, 2011. The theme of the lectures was 'Healthcare in Chaos: Models in Conflict'. Those lectures form the foundation of this book.

This book is critical of many aspects of our healthcare systems. However, despite the problems, we must bear in mind that these systems are so often staffed by thousands and thousands of idealistic and committed people, who give far more than is expected of them. It is hoped that this book may assist them in their struggles to improve their services to patients.

CHAPTER I

Power and Complexity of Culture
Healthcare Insights

Culture...educates the emotions... It consists...of implicit and often unnoticed messages about how to feel, how to respond, how to divine meaning.

(David Brooks)[1]

This chapter explains:

- ⊙ the meaning of culture and its constituent qualities: symbol, myth and ritual
- ⊙ how myths are the emotional glue that holds cultures together
- ⊙ that people apply myths to their daily experiences through narratives
- ⊙ that the founding myths of healthcare can be manipulated in ways that are contrary to their original meanings
- ⊙ through a series of praxis-oriented guidelines, the importance of a correct understanding of culture in analysing and reforming healthcare systems.

The word 'culture' is immensely popular in contemporary management textbooks, though it is rarely defined accurately. Yet the inability to appreciate the power and complexity of culture is the primary reason most organizational changes in healthcare institutions fail.[2] Culture is the missing component in the minds of planners and leaders of change. The purpose of this chapter, therefore, is to define

---

1   David Brooks (2011) *The Social Animal: The Hidden Sources of Love, Character, and Achievement.* New York: Random House, p.149.
2   Estimates of the number of changes that fail due to the neglect of cultural issues can range 'from as high as 70 or 80 per cent of all initiatives'. Mike Oram and Richard S. Wellins (1995) *Re-Engineering's Missing Ingredient: The Human Factor.* London: Institute of Personnel and Development, p.4.

the term 'culture' and demonstrate the power and complexity of culture according to contemporary thinking in social anthropology. There will be an initial analysis of a working definition of culture, to be followed by a series of guidelines that further explain its meaning. All subsequent chapters will draw on the theoretical reflections of this chapter.

An ancient Oriental fable illustrates the unsuspected dangers that await people who ignore culture. Once upon a time a monkey and a fish were in a huge flood. The agile monkey was able to save itself by grasping a tree branch and pulling itself to safety. Happy at last, the monkey noticed a fish fighting against the massive current and, deeply moved by its plight, he bent down to save it. The fish, far from happy, bit the monkey's hand, whereupon the monkey, being terribly annoyed at the fish's ingratitude, threw the fish back into the water.[3] As the water is to the fish, so culture is to the human person, a truth so difficult to grasp unless, like the fish, we experience the trauma of suddenly being deprived of a culture, a sense of belonging. Culture is a 'silent language'.[4] Cultural traditions, values, attitudes and prejudices are silent, like the stillness of water for fish, in the sense that people are most often unconscious of their presence and influence.

Defining culture

When it comes to defining more accurately the meaning of culture, however, we enter an arena of confusion. It is a popular buzzword applied to all kinds of situations; for example, we read of 'fashion culture', 'gun culture', 'corporate culture', 'internet culture' and so forth but the word remains undefined. One important document alone from the Department of Health in London, speaks of 'the culture of waiting',[5] 'a culture of reporting',[6] 'every care setting will encourage the culture',[7] 'continuing to drive a culture of greater

---

3   See D. Adams (1960) 'The monkey and the fish: Cultural pitfalls of an educational adviser.' *International Development Review 2*, 2, 22–24.

4   See Edward T. Hall (1959) *The Silent Language.* New York: Doubleday/Anchor.

5   Department of Health (2004) *The NHS Improvement Plan: Putting People at the Heart of Public Services.* London: Stationery Office, p.11.

6   Ibid., p.21.

7   Ibid., p.27.

patient safety',[8] 'a culture responsive to change'.[9] What perplexity! I sympathize with Raymond Williams' frustration: 'I don't know how many times I've wished that I'd never heard the damned word.'[10] However, despite the controversies surrounding the word culture, anthropologists agree that, as anthropologist Clifford Geertz writes, although the term is 'a deeply compromised idea', we 'cannot yet do without it'.[11] I agree with this and also with Edgar Schein, the well-known social organizational psychologist, when he writes that although culture is complex and difficult to understand, the effort 'is worthwhile because much of the mysterious and irrational in organizations suddenly becomes clear when we do understand it'.[12]

I will first present and explain a general, contemporary working definition of culture.

DEFINITION

Culture is a pattern of meanings, embedded in a network of symbols, myths, narratives and rituals that are created by individuals; a culture contains subdivisions, as people and groups struggle to respond to the competitive pressures of power and limited resources in a rapidly globalizing and fragmenting world. It instructs its adherents about what is considered to be the correct way to feel, think and behave.[13]

This definition has several advantages. First, it stresses that cultures are not entities frozen in time, without internal conflict, closed to outside forces, but processes in which people toil to find meaning in an ever-changing and often threatening environment of limited resources. Second, it emphasizes that a culture shapes people's emotional responses to the world around them. It infuses the deepest recesses of the human group, and of individuals, especially their feelings.

8   Ibid., p.31.
9   Ibid., p.63.
10   Raymond Williams (1979) *Politics and Letters: Interviews with New Left Review*. London: New Left Books, p.125.
11   Clifford Geertz (1995) *After the Fact*. Cambridge, MA: Harvard University Press, p.43.
12   Schein (1985) *Organizational Culture and Leadership*. San Francisco: Jossey-Bass, p.5.
13   See Gerald A. Arbuckle (2010) *Culture, Inculturation, and Theologians: A Postmodern Critique*. Collegeville, MN: Liturgical Press, p.17.

Raymond Williams even defines a culture as a 'structure of feeling'.[14] For this reason the common definition that a culture is primarily 'what people *do* around here' is too naively superficial. Rather a culture is 'what people *feel* about what they do'. The comment by psychoanalyst Erich Fromm is particularly incisive. The 'fact that ideas have an emotional matrix' is 'of the utmost importance' as this is 'the key to the understanding…the spirit of a culture'.[15] Schein's popular definition of organizational culture[16] unfortunately does not emphasize culture as a process, nor the element of the struggle for meaning and power through symbols, myths and rituals. Positively it does stress culture's role in forming people how to perceive, think and feel in relation to problems around them. The retelling of a simple personal event, however, will lay the first foundation for further clarifying the term.

CASE STUDY: CULTURE

In 1972 I had spent several days struggling along a dangerous narrow jungle path in the Southern Highlands of Papua New Guinea. I was weary, soaked to the skin in constant heavy rain, with little nourishing food, bitten by mosquitoes, frightened of standing on a deadly snake, constantly fearful of slipping over massive cliffs to my death below. To make matters worse, I could not speak the local language. Little wonder that I was in a depressed mood, wondering why I had agreed to trek into unknown territory. Finally I stumbled into a clearing. In the distance I noticed in the midst of mist and rain clouds a small village health clinic over which flapped a damp New Zealand flag.

Suddenly, I felt transformed. My depression disappeared. The flag evoked wonderful memories of my home in New Zealand, my family and my friends. Then stories began to emerge from deep down in my memory about the creativity and bravery of New Zealanders in chaotic times. These stories energized me. I would find a way to continue my journey, no matter how treacherous the terrain. On arrival at the little

---

14   Raymond Williams (1961) *The Long Revolution.* London: Chatto and Windus, p.41.

15   Erich Fromm (1960) *The Fear of Freedom.* London: Routledge & Kegan Paul, p.240.

16   Schein's definition of culture is: 'a pattern of basic assumptions – invented, discovered, or developed by a given group as it learns to cope with its problems of external adaption and internal integration – that has worked well enough to be considered valid and, therefore, to be taught to new members as the correct way to perceive, think, and feel in relation to those problems'. See Schein 1995, p.9.

clinic I met a group of healthcare volunteers from New Zealand who had come to one of the most isolated parts of the world to help sick people. No other clinic existed for miles around. We chatted together for several hours, sharing stories of our lives in New Zealand and discovering that we had mutual friends. I left them thoroughly rejuvenated in body, mind and heart.

We now review the constituent elements of a culture, namely: symbols, myths and rituals.

Symbols and power

DEFINITION

A symbol, such as the New Zealand flag in the above incident, is 'any reality that by its very dynamism or power leads to (that is, makes one think about, imagine, get into contact with or reach out to) another deeper and often mysterious reality through the sharing in the dynamism of the symbol itself and without additional explanation'.[17]

A symbol has many qualities:

1. First, a symbol is multivocal, that is, it simultaneously contains many meanings. The flag evoked within me a whole range of diverse meanings, for example, the magnificent scenery of the country, my family and the school I had attended. Since one symbol can be interpreted in many different ways, it is understandable that communication between people can be a difficult experience.

2. Second, a symbol is not merely a sign. Signs just *point* to the object signified, but symbols *re*-present the object; the photograph of my father evokes the very presence of my father. The flag did not point to New Zealand 3000 miles away; rather it brought the nation alive in my imagination in

17   I am grateful to Adolfo Nicolas for this definition.

a way that gave back to me a sense of belonging when I had become depressed by the frightening rigours of the journey. It is impossible to remain dispassionate about symbols, because they speak first and foremost to people's hearts. The emotive, stirring to action power of symbols, is their essential quality. Because of this affective quality, symbols have the ability to hold people's allegiance over a very long period of time. For this reason we can speak of symbols as timeless. In brief, symbols have emotional meanings. Signs are about visible experiences that can be readily quantifiable but symbols seek to move us well beyond the visible to an elevated experiential level of knowledge.

3. Third, a symbol has the ability to attract meanings around two poles, one emotional and the other cognitive. Thus not only did the New Zealand flag evoke strong feelings within me but it also reminded me of my rights as a citizen and the obligation of my government to respect them.

4. Fourth, a symbol can contain simultaneously opposite meanings. For example, the flag gave rise to an inner joy as I recalled the good experiences of being a New Zealander, but it also evoked a sense of sadness because I still would not see my family and friends in New Zealand for a long time. A stethoscope symbolizes an important diagnostic instrument, but it can simultaneously be for the patient a symbol of the superior, fear-evoking power of the clinician.

5. Fifth, there are many types of symbols, for example, structural and antistructural. The former are those that reflect the ordinary, everyday life of rules or status. To facilitate the smooth running of society, people need to know the roles individuals play. For example, I need to know that a person is a medical doctor, not a butcher, so I expect symbols outside a surgery clearly indicating that person's official role in society. Another example is the distinction between the symbols of power and powerlessness. I was once being driven in the passenger's seat of a police car with its siren and lights flashing to lecture to a group of officers. The traffic became very orderly and cars ahead of us slowed down or stopped.

To my embarrassment I rather enjoyed the chance to sit right inside a power or authority symbol, watching people scatter to let us pass by. They felt powerless in the presence of such a dominant cultural symbol.

On the other hand, there are periods in daily life in which structural roles in society become deliberately unimportant. No matter who is in a hospital as a patient – politician, doctor, lawyer, cleaner, teacher – all are equal. Societal roles are deliberately stripped away and this is achieved through the antistructural symbol 'patient'.[18]

CASE STUDIES: SYMBOLS AND POWER

I once heard of a CEO (Chief Executive Officer) of a hospital who let it be known that his office door would always be open to listen to his managers, but he failed to create symbols of openness. Rather, managers were put off by two symbols of dominant power: his domineering personal assistant at the entrance to his office and his refusal to speak to managers other than from behind his over-sized desk. Managers were made to feel powerless in the presence of the CEO.

By contrast, I recently sat in the foyer of a busy Sydney hospital watching people approach the reception desk at the emergency ward. Despite the queues of often deeply anxious people the receptionists remained immensely kind to each person. Often they would leave their desks to be closer to people who looked especially worried; I could see the immense relief on the faces of potential patients. By their behaviour the receptionists symbolized fundamental healthcare values of respect and compassion and potential patients no longer felt afraid and powerless.

6. Sixth, the meanings of symbols can change, sometimes dramatically so. In the United States medical practitioners traditionally enjoyed high social status and were commonly idealized as self-sacrificing professionals. Once healthcare

---

18   The word 'patient' is itself not a neutral symbol. For some it connotes that they should be overly submissive to the superior knowledge of a doctor; hence, the word 'consumer' is used instead. However, 'consumer' is also not without its drawbacks, because it can suggest that healthcare is primarily a business.

became defined in business terms the symbolic meaning of physician dramatically changed. In fact, by the mid-1980s 'the medical profession lost support faster than any other professional group'.[19] Professional medical work became increasingly defined as an ordinary commercial activity, more so because by '1990, physicians' fees for procedures were approximately 234% higher in the United States than in Canada, and their take-home pay was more than 50% higher than that received by Canadian doctors'.[20]

In summary, thinking symbolically is not pure rational reasoning. Nor is it fully conscious thought. Hence, it is difficult at times to be precise about the many meanings of symbols. It is difficult enough grasping the meanings of symbols used by oneself and by one's culture, but it is even more hazardous assigning meanings to symbols used by people of other cultures. Therefore, clinicians when relating to patients from cultures or ethnic groups other than their own must have considerable patience. Even with the help of official interpreters it can be difficult to fathom the meaning of the symbols being used by patients from other cultures.

Myths: Narrative symbols

Myths and mythologies (collections of interrelated myths) anthropologically are narrative symbols, that is, they are emotionally charged stories that draw people together at the deepest level of group life, and which they live by and for. Myths are value-impregnated beliefs that hold a society together, even though people may not be aware of this. Unfortunately myths are popularly assumed to be fairy tales or untruths. On the contrary, myths from an anthropological perspective are stories that claim to articulate, in an imaginative way, a fundamental truth about human life. This truth is considered as authoritative by those who accept it. Without myths people do not have any reason to be or to act. Myths differ from paradigms. The

---

19   Theodore Marmor (2004) *Fads in Medical Care, Management and Policy*. London: Nuffield Trust, p.4.
20   Ibid.

latter are *cognitive* frameworks created to describe in a comprehensible way complex realities; unlike myths they lack any emotive quality.[21] Mythologies respond to four basic human needs:

1. A *legitimating reason for existence*, that is, a need to find some satisfying reason for why things exist. For example, the statement that the hospital down the road exists to provide healing services. Structural or organizational change that is not legitimated by a people's mythology cannot succeed (see Chapter 6).

2. A *coherent cosmology*, that is, an explanation of where we fit in a comprehensible and safe world. I know, from what people say, that this hospital provides a safe healing environment in case I need to be admitted. This relieves my anxieties. In the creation mythology of the United States, the Great Seal of the nation which is copied on one side of the one-dollar bill reminds Americans that God, or some extraordinary destiny, calls them to participate in a new biblical Exodus, a new journey from the poverty and oppression of other nations, in order to join in the building of a new promised land. This mythology gives meaning to the lives of Americans by fitting them into a coherent cosmology. Every American politician who wishes to win power must legitimize their policies by reference to this creation mythology in some way or other. Such was the gift of people like Ronald Reagan and Bill Clinton.

3. A *social organization*, that is, a framework which allows us to work together in some degree of harmony and thus avoid chaos. There are clear symbols inside the hospital directing patients where they should go; this evokes in me the feeling that the organization is rightly structured to provide good services.

4. An *inspirational vision*, that is, an overall view that inculcates a sense of pride and belonging. As I enter the foyer of my hospital, I feel inspired to see staff members so approachable and caring. I feel proud that my suburb has the best hospital in the city and I want to do everything I can as a volunteer

---

21   See Jenny Stewart (2009) *Public Policy Values*. Basingstoke: Palgrave Macmillan, p.192.

to maintain this.[22] Sociologist Peter Berger comments on this quality of inspiration. Myths, he writes, have the power to lift people 'above their captivity in the ordinary, and attain powerful visions of the future, and become capable of collective actions to realize such visions'. A myth has the ability to transcend 'both pragmatic and theoretical rationality, while at the same time it strongly affects them'.[23]

By mythically defining and structuring the world, the human person and group are able to grasp to some degree or other the regions beyond human control which influence well-being and destiny. Like sacred icons, myths are the medium of revelation handed down from the heroes of the past,[24] so they are not to be lightly discarded or questioned. Like all symbols, myths can evoke deep emotional responses. No matter how committed we are to deepen our grasp of the meaning of myths, they still remain somewhat ambiguous and mysterious, because they attempt to express what can never be fully explained. The more we try the more we discover new and unexpected meanings in myths. All groups will have founding myths that are the ultimate binding forces of identity and hope in the future. As explained, for example, the founding myth of the United States is the new Israel born out of a new Exodus, the new 'Promised Land' where democracy will protect its citizens from the corrupting forces of monarchs and dictators.

Myths can contain or have solid foundations in historical reality. But the purposes of myths and history differ. History is about a succession of events, but myths evaluate their moral significance. Thus, Bill Gates, one of the best-known entrepreneurs of the personal computer age, was born in Seattle in 1955. From the historical perspective, he is described as fitting into a definite time period, influencing and being influenced by what is happening around him. If, however, he is evaluated as a person who exemplifies remarkably creative, entrepreneurial skills, the ability to amass wealth and philanthropic generosity, then we are measuring him by the founding mythology of the American nation. It is a historical fact that Alexander Fleming,

---

22   See Joseph Campbell (1970) *The Masks of God*, 4 vols. New York: Viking Press.
23   Peter Berger (1974) *Pyramids of Sacrifice: Political Ethics and Social Change.* Harmondsworth: Penguin, p.32.
24   See Thomas Fawcett (1970) *The Symbolic Language of Religion.* London: SCM Press, p.101.

a Scottish biologist and pharmacologist, discovered penicillin. From a mythological perspective, however, he fits the image of a no-nonsense, hardworking, unpretentious Scotsman.

Reservoirs of memory

Myths are symbols in narrative form that reaffirm identities. The New Zealand flag on top of the ramshackle health clinic in the jungle clearing restored my feelings of belonging, but it also evoked in me an awareness of the founding of my nation – the incredible navigation skills of the Maori peoples centuries ago as they voyaged over thousands of miles of dangerous seas, and of my ancestors from Britain and Ireland who developed a brilliant agricultural economy in the midst of a mountainous and remote countryside in the nineteenth century. Stories of cultural heroes, like Edmund Hillary who first climbed Mount Everest, and Michael Joseph Savage who laid the foundations of the welfare state and universal healthcare in New Zealand, came back to me. They innovatively triumphed with limited resources over incredible obstacles. If they succeeded despite the natural and political barriers so could I!

Not only are myths able to inculcate a sense of pride, energy, direction, or simply an *esprit de corps*, they are also reservoirs of memory and identity that people can draw on to face the challenges of life. Rollo May writes that 'myths are like the beams in a house: not exposed to outside view, they are the structure which holds the house together so people can live in it.'[25] Or they can be likened to the information concealed in the DNA of a cell, or the programme technology of a computer. A myth is the cultural DNA, the software, the unconscious information, the programme that controls the way we picture the world around us and in consequence act.

Among the many types of myths three are particularly relevant here:

1. A *public* myth is a set of stated ideals that people openly claim bind them together, for example, the mission statement of a hospital. In practice these ideals may have little or no cohesive force. One study of mission statements in surveys of

---

25   Rollo May (1991) *The Cry for Myth*. New York: Delta, p.15.

a sample of hospitals in the United States discovered that most managers 'did not perceive a high level of commitment to the statement by employees or that individual actions were very much influenced by the mission.'[26]

2. An *operative* myth is what actually gives people their felt sense of identity; the operative myth can and often does differ dramatically from the public myth.

3. A *residual* myth is one with little or no daily impact on a group's life, but which, at times, can become a very powerful operative myth.

Residual myths: Examples

○ The late Slobodan Milosevic, the Serb leader, swayed Serbian public opinion in his fiery speech of 28 June 1989 when he invoked the residual myth of humiliation that had remained dormant for centuries: Yugoslavia belonged to Serbs, he argued, despite the fact that they had been defeated in Kosovo by Muslims on 28 June 1389, and retribution for 600 years of subjugation had now to be sought in bloody warfare. The memory of the same defeat had inspired a Serb in 1914 to assassinate Archduke Franz Ferdinand of Austria, so beginning the First World War and resulting in the death of millions of people.[27]

○ A powerful residual myth came to the surface in Britain during the Falklands War. Britain had become 'great' in the past because it had learned to 'rule the waves' and establish history's largest empire. However, since 1945, with its empire disbanded, it had been reduced to a second-rate power. The Falklands War, under the leadership of Prime Minister Margaret Thatcher, offered the people the rare chance briefly of returning to the sacred time of their creation out of chaos, when a giant navy made Britain *the* world power, as Winston Churchill did in the Second World War. The sight of the ships

---

26 Duncan *et al.* 1995, p.177.
27 See Chris Hann (2000) *Social Anthropology.* Abingdon: Teach Yourself, p.141; 'Nations and their past.' (1996) *The Economist* (21 December), p.73.

sailing south to do battle became a revitalizing ritual giving the British a renewed sense of meaning and national pride.

○ On a more positive note, the residual myth of the world-class public hospital St Vincent's in the heart of Sydney, Australia's gay area, is that it was founded in 1857 by three Irish religious sisters who braved enormous difficulties primarily to serve the poor. In the 1990s, when the government threatened to close it, this residual myth surfaced in the public discourse. It so galvanized local support that the government was forced to rescind its decision. I will argue in Chapter 2 that, in Western society, it is the well-known Good Samaritan story, with its values of solidarity, equity and compassion, that is the ultimate residual myth of all contemporary public and private healthcare. The story has immense residual power to inspire people to act for society's less advantaged members.

Myths and values

Values are deeply embedded in myths. Values are action-oriented priorities, that is, they are constant and lasting beliefs shared by members of a culture about what they consider to be good or desirable or not. Values mould and shape our behaviour in our everyday life, often in an unconscious manner.[28] In the New Zealand mythology that so influenced and energized my behaviour in the jungle of Papua New Guinea, the dominant values were courage and creativity when times are tough. Yet values can be in conflict with one another and people can even have different interpretations of their meaning. This is increasingly so, for example, when the government in England insists that key values of the NHS are simultaneously equity and choice. The more the latter is emphasized, the more the financially comfortable benefit to the disadvantage of the poorer sections of the population.[29] In Canada most stakeholders accept that values in the founding story of their universal healthcare drive policy decisions and behaviour, but do not agree which values are the most important, or even precisely what they mean.

---

28   See Simon Dolan, Salvador Garcia and Bonnie Richley (2006) *Managing by Values.* Basingstoke: Palgrave Macmillan, pp.27–49.

29   See Pollock 2005, p.83.

Myth management

New myths are created and old ones maintained, constantly revised or lost completely because of a varied flow of forces, changing needs and new ways of seeing things. The creation, revision or disappearance of myths is called *myth management, which* occurs through such processes as myth revision, substitution, drift and revitalization.

Myth revision

When people scour the past to find legitimacy for an uncritical acceptance of the status quo myth revision can occur. The mythology of the United States, as mentioned above, is rooted in the belief that Americans are building the new 'Promised Land' of peace, plenty and justice for all. This accounted for the constant reference to 'the American Dream' by a wide variety of people seeking to justify retaining the healthcare status quo. They overlooked the facts that, without reforms, there was to be no promised land ahead for the millions of people who are poor and have no healthcare insurance.

Sometimes revision takes place if only the *meaning* of specific myths, not the words themselves, are changed. When the founding myth of the United States evolved it was stated in the Declaration of Independence that 'all men [*sic*] are created equal', but this equality did not include African Americans and women. For example, the medical profession was closed to them. As community standards changed so did the meaning of equality extend to these groups. Likewise there was a time when people with mental problems were blamed for their behaviour and were thus socially ostracized and institutionalized alongside criminals and paupers. Now the mythology of healthcare, while still retaining the expression 'mental problems', wisely views such people's condition as a consequence of a complex interaction of psychological, genetic/biological and socioeconomic factors. This is also reflected in the increasing use of the term mental 'diseases' rather than mental 'problems'.

Myth substitution

Myth substitution is a difficult and often painful process. For example, the official title of North Korea is the Democratic People's

Republic of Korea. Following the Second World War, which ended Japan's colonial rule of Korea, most Koreans wished for an authentic form of democracy that would guarantee political freedom. This did not happen. Communists deliberately manipulated the word 'democratic', which came to mean authoritarian oppression, and imposed this meaning on the people in the North. This is an example of an attempt to replace one myth with another, although all the while retaining the same word 'democratic'.

In England, successive governments since the mid-1980s have consciously and systematically tried to impose a new healthcare myth on their citizens, a myth no longer of universal healthcare based on the values such as equity, solidarity and justice. In its place they have sought, and continue to seek, to substitute this myth with one whose values are diametrically opposed, namely values of competition and choice.[30] In this market model of healthcare people are considered to be commodities (see Chapter 2). Yet, at the same time, the government is proclaiming it is true to the founding story of the NHS. Patricia Hewitt, as Secretary of State for Health in 2005, while publicly defending the founding values of comprehensiveness, universality and equity, was, in fact, at the same time vigorously promoting a market model of healthcare based on consumer choice, a multiplicity of competing providers.[31] Hewitt tried to justify her policies by proclaiming that they were the best way to maintain the traditional values of the NHS in a rapidly changing world.

Myth drift

Drift occurs when myths change, degenerate or disappear without most people being aware of what is happening. They assume things are as they have always been. Sometimes the dominant myth is distorted because a secondary myth assumes an exaggerated position. This has certainly happened in healthcare in England. The business aspect of healthcare has come to dominate discussions on the future of the NHS, as is the case in the United States (see Chapter 2), that

---

30 See relevant comments by Chris Shore and Susan Wright (2000) 'Coercive Accountability.' In Marilyn Strathern (ed.) *Audit Cultures: Anthropological Studies in Accountability, Ethics, and the Academy.* London: Routledge.

31 See Rudolf Klein (2006) *The New Politics of the NHS: From Creation to Reinvention,* 5th edn. Abingdon: Radcliffe Publishing, p.218.

is, the values of market efficiency and competition are emphasized at the expense of solidarity and equity. Many citizens are not aware that this drift is taking place.

Myth revitalization and heroes

Myths can speak about how chaos became cosmos, that is, an orderly world. When a people are threatened with, or experience, cultural chaos, they may feel the need to rediscover their original creation myth that gave them a sense of order. In re-articulating this myth, people are re-energized and determined to protect the founding story. For example, any attempt by politicians in Canada to undermine the myth of universal healthcare is sure to evoke strong popular criticism. The vociferous reactions of citizens revitalize the proud founding story, namely that all Canadians must have reasonable access to health services freed from financial costs to themselves. The retelling of the story gives people the renewed energy to resist efforts to change it.

There are three key factors in revitalization: first, a feeling of cultural confusion or chaos; second, the emergence of cultural heroines or heroes who are in touch with the culture's founding myths; and, third, the willingness of people to participate in the reliving or reappropriation of the founding story. The myth can be updated, distorted or purified in the process. Myths frequently recount incidents of exemplary individuals whose manner of living shows how the mythical values of the culture are to be expressed. These heroes and heroines venture out into the unknown world, where they battle against evil and articulate the tensions we feel, for example, the tension that exists between society and the individual. They show how the forces of chaos and evil can be kept at bay and tensions resolved in a culturally acceptable manner. Reflect on my own story of being re-energized in the jungle in Papua New Guinea by the example of New Zealand cultural heroes.

REVITALIZATION OF MYTHS: EXAMPLES

In American Western films, as in *Shane* (1953) or *Cat Ballou* (1965), the hero is a strong, self-contained individual unknown to or not fully accepted by society, who possesses exceptional abilities he uses successfully to defend a powerless society against the evil actions of the villain. The society finally accepts the saviour it had earlier rejected. The cowboy hero of Western films has now been modernized through the *Rocky* and *Rambo* films of Sylvester Stallone and, in more recent times, through the *Terminator* films of Arnold Schwarzenegger. The vigorously individualistic, macho, physically strong, thoroughly self-contained and silent person, the 'truly American' hero, is centre stage once more, destroying villains with modern firepower, using helicopters in place of horses, restoring the morale of the American people, prepared to return at any time when needed to uphold the American way of life. However, in the light of heroes like George Washington and Abraham Lincoln, these updated versions of the mythic hero are a distortion of what the hero should be, because of the senseless use of violence.

The founding heroes of the NHS in Britain are William Beveridge, Aneurin Bevan as Minister of Health, and Prime Minister Clement Attlee. Particularly under Bevan's direction the National Health Service Act of 1948 was passed, providing everyone with free diagnosis and treatment of illness, at home or in hospital, as well as dental and ophthalmic services. Subsequent politicians, especially Margaret Thatcher and Tony Blair, have become mythic heroes to many in Britain, but they have in fact distorted the founding story with their plans to gradually corporatize and privatize healthcare services (a point more fully explained in Chapter 2).

Ritual

> DEFINITION
>
> Ritual is the repetitive spontaneous or prescribed symbolic use of bodily movement and gesture to express and articulate meaning within a social context in which there is possible or real tension/conflict and a need to resolve or hide it.[32]

Ritual is among the most basic, frequent and important of human actions. In fact, without ritual we cannot remain human for we would be unable to communicate with one another. Through ritual we give flesh to the values and goals expressed in myths. Take the simple act of shaking hands. According to Western custom, when people resolve or hide a tension/conflict between them, they shake hands. It is a gesture of stylized form that, outwardly at least, conveys the meaning that peace has been restored. If I refuse to shake the hand of someone I am sending the dangerous message that he or she is an enemy. Following a football match it is customary for both teams to shake hands. The defeated team may be extremely angry with the victors, but the ritual will hide this. The shaking of hands by opposing players is a ritual visibly expressing a fundamental myth of sport that, despite the mutual aggression during play, 'it is only a game'.

All social life moves on a continuum between two possible poles: absolute order and absolute spontaneity/chaos. There is an ongoing tension between these extremes, with consequent uncertainty and fear, which needs to be controlled in some visible form. The greater the tension in relationships, the more urgent it is to develop rituals that ease the anxieties. Ritual brings order out of chaos. Because people's health and well-being are involved it is not surprising that many detailed rituals must be formulated and adhered to in healthcare institutions. These rituals seek to bring anxieties under control. For example, the process of becoming a patient in a hospital normally evokes anxieties of the unknown. Hence, there are orderly rituals that aim to allay these fears, such as specialized staff who guide patients

---

32   See Robert Bocock (1974) *Ritual in Industrial Society: A Sociological Analysis of Ritualism in Modern England.* London: George Allen and Unwin, pp.35–59, and Arbuckle 2010, pp.82–98.

through the reading and signing of documents, placing personal belongings in secure places, wheeling them to the appropriate ward. Without these rituals of formally entering a hospital a patient's anxieties intensify, even possibly further endangering their health.

CASE STUDY: RITUAL

The hand-washing by clinicians before and after seeing a patient is a crucial ritual; it is a visible expression of hospital mythology that places the welfare of the patient as its paramount concern. However, a 2008 report on acute care services in public hospitals in New South Wales, Australia, severely criticized clinicians, especially doctors, for 'spreading infections from patient to patient largely because they do not practise hand hygiene before and after seeing each patient'.[33] Over half the doctors failed to wash their hands before and after seeing each patient. Following the report's reprimand of doctors, the health department set out, in detail, the ritual that must be followed, namely 'Five Moments for Hand Hygiene': before touching a patient; before a procedure; after a procedure or body fluid exposure risk; after touching a patient; and after touching a patient's surroundings.[34] It warned clinicians that failures to adhere to the ritual would result in severe penalties.

It will be clear from the above analysis that the word 'culture' is an exceedingly complex one. Culture is a system of social interaction through shared symbols and meanings. This symbolic action must be interpreted, read or translated in order to be comprehended. Hence, real-life social action of individuals, including their feelings, can never be ignored in any study of organizational cultures. Clifford Geertz says that we are suspended in webs of significance we ourselves have spun, and culture is these webs. We cannot speak of people 'having a culture', because we exist in the midst of, use and create a world of cultural symbols.[35]

---

33 Peter Garling (2008b) *Final Report of the Special Commission of Inquiry: Acute Care Services in NSW Public Hospitals: Overview.* Sydney: NSW Government, p.16.
34 See NSW Independent Panel (2010b) *Independent Panel: Caring Together: The Health Action Plan for NSW – Third Progress Report November 2010.* Sydney: NSW Independent Panel, p.30.
35 See Clifford Geertz (1973) *The Interpretation of Cultures.* New York: Basic Books, pp.4–6.

Culture: Practical guidelines for healthcare

Since no one definition can possibly embrace all the multifaceted realities of culture, it is helpful to highlight particular facets of the concept of culture in the form of general practical interconnected guidelines that are relevant to healthcare institutions staff. This will help staff members to appreciate better why the above theory has realistic consequences for relating to one another, to their organizational system and to patients. These guidelines will be further explained and particular applications will be suggested in subsequent chapters.[36]

Guideline 1: A culture is not homogeneous, but highly fragmented into a diversity of subcultures, such as are found in healthcare systems

The term *subcultures* refers to groups within a larger culture that symbolically define themselves, or are defined by others, in opposition to the majority. More particularly, a subculture is a method of defining and honouring the particular design and identity of different interests of a group of people within a larger collectivity. Thus subcultures consist of people, in tight or loosely connected groupings, who:

- share some common interests, values, tastes and often specialist knowledge and linguistic jargon
- adhere to the same rituals and pastimes to some degree or other.

The term subculture is particularly postmodern for it is a reminder that cultures are not homogeneous, but highly fragmented.[37] In every subculture, there is always an element, sometimes strongly evident, of protest against the dominant culture of which it is part and/or against other competing subcultures. The more that people of the subculture feel threatened by the dominant group, the stronger and more vivid will be their symbols of protest and resistance.

---

36   See Gerald A. Arbuckle (2004) *Violence, Society, and the Church: A Cultural Approach*. Collegeville, MN: Liturgical Press, pp.15–27.

37   See Peter Brooker (1999) *A Concise Glossary of Cultural Theory*. London: Arnold, pp.208–209.

No hospital is a neatly integrated culture. Rather, it is an uneasy coalition of multiple subcultures, each competing for power in order to acquire control over limited resources. David Hunter, commenting on the NHS in Britain, makes the same point. He writes that the NHS is similar 'to a huge arena in which the various groups play out their power struggles'. He concludes that 'for all practical purposes each profession in the NHS behaves according to its own particular core values and beliefs'.[38] Subcultures that are not politically astute are severely handicapped in their efforts to maintain or acquire control over scarce resources. The subculture of medical clinicians, in contrast to those of nurses and other healthcare workers, has cultivated over many years political skills to maintain and develop their status and financial rewards. No government, for example, has been able to introduce universal healthcare without lengthy and conflicting negotiations with politically powerful medical subcultures.[39]

Guideline 2: Groups see their culture/subculture as 'clean' or 'pure' and others as 'dirty' or 'impure', and therefore dangerous – to be avoided, changed or eliminated

Relations between different subcultures in hospitals, for example, medical clinicians, nurses, pharmacists, radiographers, laboratory researchers and physiotherapists, are often strained because of a lack of mutual understanding and respect.[40] Yet there is a cultural factor that encourages this inter-subcultural tension. Through symbols, myths and rituals cultures and subcultures have an inbuilt tendency to create boundaries with powerful feelings like 'us and them', that is 'they' are not as good as 'we' are! The English poet Rudyard Kipling describes ethnocentrism in this way: 'All nice people, like Us are We, and everyone else is They.'[41]

---

38   Hunter 2002, pp.61–62.
39   See Klein 2006, pp.17–19.
40   See David Blane (1997) 'Health Professions.' In Graham Scambler (ed.) *Sociology as Applied to Medicine*, 4th edn. London: W.B. Saunders.
41   Rudyard Kipling (1926) 'We and They.' *Debits and Credits*. London: Macmillan, pp.327–328.

'WE/THEY' DYNAMIC IN HEALTHCARE

The profession of medical clinicians has long been dominant in healthcare. However, in recent times nurses, as a subculture, have become increasingly academically qualified. Their expertise and hands-on experience mean that they could well be doing an increasing amount of work normally undertaken by medical clinicians. But this 'intrusion' into their field of expertise is frequently vigorously resisted by medical clinicians.[42] In Britain, women, comprising most of the nursing workforce, still suffer inequality of job opportunity, low status positions and poor pay within the healthcare service, despite the fact that they make up over two-thirds of the workforce.

It is not surprising, therefore, that, as long as nurses are excluded from collaborating with medical clinicians in governance in ways that respect their expertise, there is a worldwide decline in the nursing workforce numbers. Hospitals are thus compelled to employ temporary staff unfamiliar with a ward's rituals, who may be directed to different wards each day. The quality of patient care is bound to suffer. In Australia women as specialists are still generally confined to certain tasks thought to be 'women's work', such as gynaecology, paediatrics or plastic surgery, though this is slowly changing as more and more women are graduating as doctors. In fact, over the last 30 years the percentage of women graduating from medical schools has been higher than men. Even within the medical profession itself there are 'we/they' status divisions. Hospital consultants, particularly those in specialist occupations such as cardiology and neurosurgery, have higher status than medical clinicians involved with the care of the elderly, the mentally ill, the chronically sick and public health.

Anthropologist Mary Douglas' explanation helps to throw some further light on status divisions in healthcare and the obstacles people face as they attempt upward mobility. She focuses on a

---

42   See Evan Willis (1994) *Illness and Social Relations: Issues in the Sociology of Health Care.* St Leonards: Allen and Unwin, pp.17–18.

people's understanding of 'purity' and 'pollution'.[43] For Douglas, when explaining her understanding of pollution, the object of our deepest anxieties is everyday dirt. It evokes an attitude, 'ugh!', and demands a response, 'this must be cleaned up!' What is considered dirty in some way or other pollutes or defiles what is clean and must be put aside. An appreciation of what causes things to be called dirty or clean, Douglas argues, may uncover the deepest mysteries of the moral order itself, the reasons that some societies renew and reaffirm their fundamental collective feelings and beliefs, while others do not even bother.[44]

The question is – why are things considered dirty and other things clean? Why are shoes judged dirty when placed on the table, but clean when on the floor? It is the location that defines their dirtiness and its power to evoke a reaction. As Douglas writes: 'Dirt is the by-product of a systematic ordering and classification of matter, in so far as ordering involves rejecting inappropriate elements.'[45] This means that what is thought to be dirty is relative. Douglas comments: 'It's a relative idea. Shoes are not dirty in themselves, but it is dirty to place them on the dining-table;…it is dirty to leave cooking utensils in the bedroom;…out-of-door things downstairs… In short, our pollution behaviour is the reaction which condemns any object or idea to confuse or contradict cherished classifications.'[46] It is not just a question of actual place that condemns something to be dirty or clean. Shoes are not dirty just because they are on the table rather than on the floor, but that they *should* be on the floor, and *not* on the table. There is a moral quality to reality that makes the matter of classification, and misclassification, also as an issue of right and wrong. When we say that shoes should not be on the floor we are not only stating a fact about 'the mechanical appropriateness of nature, but a moral evaluation of that order'.[47] The dread of pollution is like the horror people can have of immorality or sin.

Every human society and organization subscribes, mostly unconsciously, to rules of purity and pollution in some form or other.

---

43 See Mary Douglas (1966) *Purity and Danger: An Analysis of the Concepts of Pollution and Taboo*. London: Routledge & Kegan Paul.
44 See Robert Wuthnow *et al.* (1984) *Cultural Analysis*. London: Routledge & Kegan Paul, p.85.
45 Douglas 1966, p.48.
46 Ibid.
47 See Wuthnow *et al.* 1984, p.87.

A culture or subculture is a purity system – that is, it tells people what is pure and clean, or evil and therefore dangerous or polluting. The fear of pollution defines and protects the boundaries of a group. Pollution, as opposed to purity, interferes with the acceptable equilibrium, destroys or confuses desirable boundaries, and evokes destructive forces or conditions. As Douglas writes: 'In short, our pollution behaviour is the reaction which condemns any object or idea likely to confuse or contradict cherished classifications.'[48]

Guideline 3: Cultures constrain individuals to varying degrees

Douglas has also produced stimulating thoughts on the interconnections between culture, power, ritual and cosmology.[49] She grounds her reflections on two independently varying social criteria she terms *grid* and *group* and concludes that each location on the *grid/group* model has its own cultural bias.[50] That is, it is disposed to have a worldview and pattern of values, and a specific way of resolving disputes or tensions.

By *grid* she means the set of rules according to which people relate to one another. The second variable is the *group*. This is a community's sense of identity in relationship to people beyond its boundaries. Douglas claims that cosmological ideals and the importance of ritual will differ predictably with the extent to which group and grid are stressed. The social body constrains the way the physical body is seen; thus if there are tight controls over how people are to dress and act bodily, then there will be a rigidly controlled social group and vice versa. Obedience is demanded to the social order. In an operating theatre all present must be attired in surgical clothing to maintain a germ-free environment and adhere to strictly defined rituals. No exceptions permitted.

By contrast, if social control is weak, the body is at ease, informal, untidy and sloppy as with loose-fitting clothes or unkempt hair. For example, medical staff once out of the rigid controls of the theatre

---

48 Douglas 1966, p.48.
49 See Mary Douglas (1970) *Natural Symbols: Explorations in Cosmology.* New York: Pantheon Books.
50 See Mary Douglas (1978) *Cultural Bias.* London: Royal Anthropological Institute.

are likely to relax in their common room informally dressed with the symbols of their professional identity discarded. Douglas would term this common room experience a *weak group/weak grid* culture. Douglas Davies, when commenting on Douglas' distinctions, uses contemporary colloquial language: the theatre scene is the 'uptight' culture and the common room the 'laid-back' culture. In brief the greater degree of social control a group wields over individuals the greater the extent of control individuals must exert over how people dress and act.[51] The relation of the individual to society differs with the restraints of grid and group; the more rigid the grid and group are, the more developed the idea of formal transgression and its dangerous results and the less preoccupation there is for the right of the inner self to be freely and openly expressed.[52]

Strong group/weak grid

Purity and pollution (see Guidelines 2 and 3 above) of both the human body and social body are particular worries of people who are restrained in various ways by group and grid. The breaking of purity rules produces dangers for the individual and society; the person and society become ritually 'dirty', so that there must be rituals to remove the impurity and the danger. Witch-hunting is particularly noticeable when the culture is a *strong group/weak grid* because of fear that the boundaries of the group will be attacked and broken by disparate and dangerous forces from within. Rules of purity rarely govern internal relations, and if they do there is little concern about the consequences should they be infringed. There is greater concern, however, for inner rather than outer purity. Sects or cults would fit the category *strong group/weak grid*. They are strongly egalitarian and supportive of their collective identity; they emphasize consensus and collaboration, but demonize non-members and suspect conspiracies against them, even at times from within.[53]

National health systems resemble the *strong group/weak grid* culture model. When faced with external threats to identity, for example,

---

51 Douglas J. Davies (2011) *Emotion, Identity, and Religion: Hope, Reciprocity, and Otherness.* Oxford: Oxford University Press, p.53.

52 Douglas 1970, p.102.

53 See comments by Philip Smith and Alexander Riley (2009) *Cultural Theory: An Introduction.* Oxford: Blackwell, pp.78–79.

plans by governments to reduce resources, subcultures readily unite to defend the national system. But within the system there are vigorous power movements by different subcultures to attain control over limited resources at the expense of rivals. Sometimes there are temporary alliances of subcultures to protect or gain power, but they readily break apart if a more beneficial option should emerge for a particular subculture. Some develop sect-like behaviour, refusing to collaborate with outsiders in any significant way. As will be explained in Chapter 3, medical clinicians and managers belong to rival subcultures, each behaving at times like opposing sects; individuals are demonized if they dare to participate in dialogue in a substantive way with members of the rival subculture.

Weak group/strong grid

If a culture is *weak group/strong grid* it will be characterized by a high degree of individualism and administered by impersonal exchange relations. For example, entrepreneurial capitalists have little commitment to a collective identity and assume that market forces are able to resolve social problems. However, strictly defined business rules must be followed; if not, people are legally punished and/or ostracized by their colleagues. Community nurses are also *weak group/strong grid;* they are constantly travelling to serve the needs of patients and rarely meet as a group. Hence, they have a limited loyalty to collective identity, but a strong commitment to the rules governing their work with patients.

Strong group/strong grid

In a culture that approximates to a *strong group/strong grid* model members are expected to fit into a tradition-based, hierarchical system, in which there are rigidly defined rules governing interaction. Such is the case with groups like the army, police, church and medical clinicians. People at the top are assumed to have a monopoly over knowledge. To maintain conformity there are detailed and rigid, morally sanctioned roles about how the people must act. To break these rules is to risk ritual pollution which the ritual guardians of the system alone can remove. The hierarchical leaders' task is to maintain the status quo, and for that personal charismatic qualities are not needed – in fact, they may be dangerous in drawing people away from tradition to a culture of the leader and setting precedents for undermining the status quo in the group. For example, an airline crew's culture approximates to this model. Rules are unambiguous about how individual crew members must relate to one another and to the captain who has the ultimate control. Too much is at stake to allow individual decision-making. Medical examples are, of course, the surgical team in an operating theatre referred to earlier, the team in the emergency department and the Royal College of Physicians, which began licensing physicians in London in 1518.

Biological kinship can be used as a metaphor. When people relate to one another as though they were members of a biological kinship group this extension of the idiom of kinship is termed 'fictive'. This is particularly characteristic of *strong group/strong grid* cultures, especially when their boundaries are threatened from outside. They develop a siege mentality – 'they' (i.e. the public, mass media) are 'out to get us' and 'we' must protect ourselves from attack. The combined need to maintain a strong identity and the fear of 'them' has serious consequences: first, the group can become far more concerned to preserve the system of internal rules and regulations than about their methods of relating to the public; and, second, members are tempted to hide mistakes or corrupt practices in order to maintain the loyalty of 'the brotherhood' and public goodwill. If a member does inform on a colleague he or she must be immediately ostracized.[54] Or, if a member is exposed by outsiders for malpractice, he or she is ostracized and blamed, but the internal system that allows this behaviour to occur is not often critiqued (see Chapter 6 for further explanation).

This helps to explain the examples of failures at self-regulation by the medical profession and the consequent calls in recent years for government intervention to break the culture of 'brotherhood protection' to ensure that accountability systems are in place and are operative. The distinction is made between medical failures due to 'bad apples', that is, cases that are infrequent but involve high media exposure, and 'adverse events', that is, medical errors causing harm but that are generally preventable. It was estimated in 2001

---

54   See Arbuckle 2004, pp.46, 51.

that as many as 98,000 people die annually as a result of medical errors in hospitals in the United States; more people, for example, die from medication errors than from workplace injuries.[55] Official Australian reports reveal that preventable medical error in hospitals is responsible for 11 per cent of all deaths in the country.[56] This was described recently 'as Australia's best kept secret'.[57] In addition to the human suffering due to poor accountability the financial costs are enormous. In Britain, it was estimated in 2000 that the costs to the NHS of hospital-acquired infections amounted to nearly £1 billion annually.[58] In Australia, it was estimated in 1999 that inappropriate medication use resulted in at least 80,000 hospital admissions annually at a cost of about $350 million; approximately half the admissions were considered preventable.[59] The medical profession has been particularly reluctant to acknowledge, and learn from, adverse events. Governments, responding to the need to make physicians more publicly accountable, have introduced new agencies such as the National Institute of Clinical Excellence (NICE) in Britain, the Canadian Institute for Health Information (CIHI), the Clinical Excellence Commission (CEC) and the Bureau of Health Information (BHI) in New South Wales, Australia.

Weak group/weak grid

A culture of the *weak group/weak grid* type is strongly egalitarian in social relationships and in gender, with minimum pressure from structures within and at the boundaries of the group. Generally, communities of this type emerge only under the inspiration of some charismatic leader, who denounces the oppressive rigidity of the *group/grid* traditions or structures of a dominant culture from which

---

55 See Lyn Wright *et al.* (2001) *Clinical Leadership and Clinical Governance: A Review of Developments in New Zealand and Internationally* (August), 18. Accessed on 30 April 2011 at www.hiirc.org.nz/assets/sm/.../CCAN2litreviewfind.pdf?download....

56 'Drugs and medical errors killing one of every five Australians' (2009) *Best Health*. Accessed 14 June 2012 at www.besthealth.com.au/drugs-and-medical-errors-killing-one-of-every-five-australians.

57 Jeff Richardson reported by Julia Medew (2011) 'Thousands dying from preventable hospital errors.' Accessed 14 June 2012 at www.theage.com.au/national/thousands-dying-from-preventable-hospital-errors-says professor.

58 For a detailed analysis see Department of Health (DoH) (2000a) *An Organisation with a Memory*. London: DoH.

59 See 'Drugs and medical errors killing one of every five Australians' 2009.

escape is sought. Dress codes and rigid rules of conduct based on tradition are considered irrelevant; far more important is the interior conversion and effective commitment of members to the group's vision and values resulting in what anthropologically are termed *intentional communities.*

I have seen this type of community several times in hospital emergency department teams. Members are committed to one thing – the saving of the lives of people in front of them; status differences within the team are of far less importance. The Jewish philosopher Martin Buber (1878–1965) defines the way in which individuals interact as the 'I–Thou' relationship. This relationship happens when there is mutuality, openness, presence and directness.[60] Anthropologist Victor Turner describes the model as a *liminality* experience. In liminality, status and roles are not the dominant force, but the fact that people are all human persons committed to search together for and live by human values. When people are in the process of liminality they are apt to experience what Turner terms *communitas*, that is, a sense of oneness with other people in which statuses and roles become of secondary importance.[61] Liminality is crucial for creativity, 'it breaks as it were, the cake of custom and enfranchises speculation'.[62] Without experiences of liminality, people lose their ability to reflect, to reimagine a world that is different; they become suffocated with the sheer weight of custom. There is government by consensus; the authority/power types within this model are predominantly personal and reciprocal, the latter being reflected in the openness of the group to new insights, dialogue and outsiders. Personal identity according to this model comes from an awareness of one's self-worth, not from a culture's traditional internal status systems and boundary structures.

Although to establish it is extremely difficult, this *weak group/weak grid* culture model as the foundation for successful teamwork is of significant importance in healthcare, requiring very skilled leadership indeed (see Chapter 5). For example, the qualities of the 'I–Thou'

---

60   See Martin Buber (2002) *Between Man and Man.* New York: Routledge, p.xii.
61   See Victor Turner (1974) *Dramas, Fields and Metaphors: Symbolic Action in Human Society.* New York: Cornell University Press, p.232.
62   Victor Turner (1967) *The Forest of Symbols: Aspects of Ndembu Rituals.* Ithaca NY: Cornell University Press, p.106.

relationship are fundamental to healing the inner pain of illness; clinicians and patients are equal people whose hearts are open to each other. Also, clinicians and administrators are prepared to experience an 'I–Thou' relationship, that is, they put aside traditional rivalries and become capable of reimagining together profoundly new ways of collaborating for the good of patients.

Guideline 4: Cultures connote power or lack of power

Power in cultures, traditionally defined as the ability to influence, takes many forms. *Position* power is the capacity to use power flowing from the status of the person in an organization, for example, a CEO has position power over a hospital complex; *coercive* power is the ability to force people to act through fear of punishment; *reward* encourages a response by offering or declining to give benefits; *personal* power is the capacity to influence because of personal/ expert qualities. In addition there is *unilateral* and *reciprocal* power. A person exercising unilateral power refuses to be influenced by others, so that dialogue is impossible; a bully exercises unilateral power (see Chapter 4). Reciprocal power, however, allows a person not only to influence others, but also to be influenced by others; this form of power is integral to all genuine dialogue and is a particular characteristic of *weak group/weak grid* cultures (see Chapter 5).

Michel Foucault: Disciplinary and surveillance power

While acknowledging these types of power, Michel Foucault (1926–1984), the French philosopher, introduces a wholly different way of understanding power in contemporary societies. He claimed to find configurations of unnecessarily coercive power relations in social situations as professions, churches, police and social welfare agencies. He associated the developing power of these organizations with the production of ever more specialized knowledge which, in turn, has been able to control more and more spheres of private life. The control is exercised by imposing classifications which result in developing progressively finer distinctions between acceptable and unacceptable ideas of a normal individual's behaviour. Categorizing people into professional groups such as doctors or religious ministers, force individuals into 'social boxes', leading society uncritically to accept this domination.

To understand Foucault's proposition that power which is ubiquitous and insidious is predominantly *disciplinary*, it is necessary to first appreciate what he means by 'discourses' and the central role of the human body in their development. For him a discourse is the organization of ideas and language that uniquely characterize every institution.[63] It is a collection of specialized knowledge through which the controlling elite is able to discipline others. Power and knowledge in discourses 'directly imply one another...there is no power relation without the correlative constitution of the field of knowledge'. He continues: 'The subject who knows, the objects to be known and the modalities of knowledge must be regarded as so many effects of these fundamental implications of power/knowledge and their historical transformations.'[64]

Foucault explains his theory with particular reference to the historical development of the discourse of the medical profession which has the capacity to define bodies as deviant or normal, as hygienic or unhygienic, as controlled or requiring control. He writes: '[Medicine] set itself up as the supreme authority in matters of hygienic necessity... [It] promised to eliminate defective individuals, degenerate and bastardized populations.' He goes further: 'In the name of biological and historical urgency, it justified the racisms of the state...it grounded them in "truth".'[65] In his book, *The Birth of the Clinic* (1975),[66] he further explains his analysis of the relationship between disciplinary power and surveillance. He speaks of the 'anatomical atlas' which is the human body formed from the medico-scientific gaze. Since medical practices altered in the late eighteenth century, the adoption of procedures as the physical examination, the post-mortem, the use of the stethoscope, psychiatry, radiology, surgery, the establishment of hospitals and doctors' surgeries, have all resulted in an ever-increasing power over the body. People are

---

63   See Michel Foucault (1979a) *Discipline and Punish: The Birth of the Prison.* Harmondsworth: Penguin, p.27.
64   Ibid., pp.27–28.
65   Michel Foucault (1979b) *The History of Sexuality, Volume 1: An Introduction.* Harmondsworth: Penguin, p.54.
66   Michel Foucault (1975) *The Birth of the Clinic: An Archaeology of Medical Perception.* New York, NY: Vintage Books.

expected to surrender authority over their bodies to the medical profession, the supreme example of surveillance. He speaks of 'strategies' of power, that is, the ways in which institutions construct forms of power and then insist that they alone can control its use. Once people are socially defined as insane then they must be controlled accordingly. People who dominate specialized disciplines hold extraordinary power in society, power that can rarely be challenged by outsiders. Power insidiously permeates every aspect of particular cultures/subcultures and is psychologically invasive and oppressive. Both agents and subjects of power are rarely aware of this subjugation.[67]

Since the eighteenth century the physical human body, he claims, has become the primary location of disciplinary political and ideological power, surveillance and regulation. With the body and its actions in mind, the structures of the state, health departments, educational systems, psychiatry, the law and others classify the limits of behaviour and document activities, disciplining those bodies which violate the established boundaries in order to make them politically and economically valuable.

According to Foucault, the surveillance power of medical knowledge is symptomatic of wider trends in the Western world. This power of surveillance and control especially resides in self-perpetuating cultural systems and individuals become their watching agents. It is this power that is intensifying in all areas of life through an ever-increasing array of laws, rules and rituals. We are ceaselessly under scrutiny by all kinds of people such as clinicians, police, security guards, bureaucrats and, in recent years, through the dramatic increase in closed circuit security television. In shops, workplaces, on highways and in all kinds of public areas, surveillance can now occur throughout the entire day and year. Even if there is no surveillance, people still think someone is watching.

---

67   See Michel Foucault (1974) *The Order of Things: An Archaeology of the Human Sciences.* New York: Vintage Books.

Guideline 5: Social networking fragments cultural boundaries

Social networking is a term that describes the process whereby individuals, within the same culture or across cultural boundaries, converse online on a casual or social basis with people they know, or do not know, but with whom they share common interests. People, through an ever-expanding process of social networking, negotiate their relationship to natural, social and economic realities in the midst of a rapidly changing, chaotic globalizing and computer-age world. Social networking is undoubtedly an increasingly dominant method of negotiating for power through information in our computerized and globalized environment. The term 'network society' was first used in the mid-1990s by sociologist Manuel Castells, who argued that the network model that operates in information technology 'provides the material basis for its pervasive expansion through the entire social structure'.[68] Networks are shaped by movements of information that undermine the usual patterns of identity based on particular physical, social, cultural and functional qualities. Castells argues that today's society is noted for its increasing polarization of networked elites in relation to those who remain outside the boundaries of global networks. In other words, network society is dominated by mobile international elites, and creates new forms of social exclusion of the stationary poor.

Social networking is already having a profound impact on healthcare. Approximately one-third of Americans who go online to research their health use social networks to find fellow patients and discuss their conditions. About 36 per cent of social network users evaluate and influence other consumers' knowledge prior to making healthcare decisions. An estimated 60 per cent of surveyed physicians and 65 per cent of surveyed nurses in the United States are interested in using social networks for professional purposes.[69]

---

68 Manuel Castells (1996) *The Power of Identity: Volume 2: The Information Age: Economy, Society and Culture.* Oxford: Blackwell, p.469.
69 See Deloitte Center for Health Solutions (2010) *Issue Brief: Social Networks in Health Care: Communication, Collaboration and Insights 1*, 4. Accessed 15 August 2011 at www.deloitte.com/centerforhealthsolutions.

Guideline 6: A culture is a process of struggling to contain chaos, yet an experience of chaos is an essential precondition for innovative action

For sociologist Peter Berger culture protects people from the awesome insecurities and meaninglessness of chaos (*anomy*), that is, the radical breakdown of order or predictability. Culture (*nomos*) is 'an area of meaning carved out of a vast mass of meaninglessness, a small clearing of lucidity in a formless, dark, almost ominous jungle'.[70] Disruptive experiences of chaos can be catalysts for radical cultural changes (see Chapter 6). To further understand their insights into *anomy* anthropologists are even applying the basic assumptions of the Chaos theory of physics to the study of cultures. Broadly defined the theory is 'the science of process rather than state, of becoming rather than being...[resulting in] a science of the global nature of systems'.[71] It means that chaos and order interact and are always on the borders of the other. The movement of change is not smooth, but lurching, and its necessary impetus is stress. At certain points, changes may amplify into disturbances so profound and deep that a culture breaks apart, but may eventually reconfigure itself into a much more complex system.[72]

As already noted in the above explanation of Turner's insight into *liminality*, chaos is a freeing or subversive experience, for it cracks the shell of custom or habit, permitting the imagination to dream of alternative or drastically different ways of acting or doing things. When people own their own chaos, admitting their powerlessness, they are able to return to the sacred time of the founding of the group. There they can ask fundamental questions about the group's origins, about what is essential to the founding vision and should be kept, and what is accidental and should be allowed to go (see Chapters 5 and 6).

---

70 Peter Berger (1969) *The Sacred Canopy: Elements of a Sociological Theory of Religion*. New York: Doubleday, p.23.
71 James Glieck (1987) *Chaos: Making a New Science*. New York: Penguin, p.5.
72 See Mark S. Mosko and Frederick H. Damon (eds) (2005) *On the Order of Chaos: Social Anthropology and the Science of Chaos*. New York: Berghahn.

CASE STUDIES: CHAOS AND INNOVATIVE CHANGE

The experience of the giant corporate cultures of IBM and AT&T in the United States exemplifies this guideline. Through government anti-trust action, AT&T had to be broken apart in 1984, much to the enjoyment of IBM. AT&T's organizational culture dissolved into chaos, IBM's did not; yet it is AT&T that eventually triumphed. It used chaos to fundamentally rethink its mission and significantly moved to rebuild itself. Its stock rose 222 per cent, with concomitant winning awards for quality, but IBM lost two-thirds of its market share.[73]

In a totally different field, there is the example of Alexander Fleming's 'accidental' discovery in 1928 of what eventually became known as penicillin. The orderly arrangement of his laboratory culture had been seriously disturbed. To make room for another scientist to experiment while he himself was on vacation, he had piled dishes into a messy pool of Lysol disinfectant. On his return to the laboratory, he found several dishes had remained above the disinfectant. While viewing one of the dishes that had escaped the cleaning he noticed that a mould had grown and it had apparently killed the *Staphylococcus aureus* that had been growing in the dish. This led Fleming eventually to conclude that the mould might have therapeutic potential.

Guideline 7: Since people fear the unknown, cultures have an in-built resistance to change, and this can lead to violence against people or groups who advocate change; cultures serve as defences against individual and group anxiety

Following Berger's insight into *nomos*, that is, culture as order or predictability, culture is a human creation that protects us from the fear-evoking dark abyss of disorder. Little wonder, writes Berger, that an innovator can become the object of violence, scapegoating or marginalization: 'The individual who strays seriously from the socially defined programs can be considered not only a fool or a knave but a madman.'[74] This is why cultural change is a profoundly

---

73 See Margorie Kelly (1993) 'Taming the demons of change.' *Business Ethics: The Magazine of Corporate Responsibility 4*, 7.

74 Berger 1969, p.23.

messy, agonizing, and uncertain process. It takes a long time for individuals to allow their hearts to accept what their heads may be telling them, that change is essential.

From experience we know that individually and corporately we so dread the pain of chaos that we often resist it. In theory we frequently proclaim we are open to change, but in practice powerful inner forces move us to resist it, even in matters of seemingly little importance. Think about how you feel when someone dares to sit in your favourite armchair in front of the television! When cultural predictability is seriously threatened or disintegrates, we can experience the darkness of meaninglessness, or the crushing taste of chaos, just as I did on the jungle path in Papua New Guinea. The poet Dante Alighieri, writing in the fourteenth century, describes chaos as 'a forest dark... So bitter is it, death is little more.'[75] Change, even at times the faintest whisper of it, substitutes ambiguity and uncertainty for the known, and we yearn for the predicable that frees us from the fear of the unknown. As management consultant Margaret Wheatley comments, 'We are not comfortable with chaos, even in our thoughts, and we want to move out of confusion as quickly as possible.'[76]

Cultures have also been defined as 'defences against anxieties', 'containers of anxieties',[77] even 'psychic prisons',[78] in an effort to describe their inner power to resist change and to bully would-be change agents into conformity. Shirley P. Lowry concludes her study of myths with the assertion: 'Most mythic systems agree on this basic point: What promotes cosmic order, harmony, and life is good, and what promotes chaos, disintegration, and death is evil.'[79] And Edgar Schein, well-known management psychologist, is realistic in assessing the possibility of cultural change. He writes that 'major cultural change usually takes a long time – 25 years in the case of

75 Dante Alighieri (1909) *The Divine Comedy*, trans. Henry W. Longfellow. New York: Doubleday, p.15.
76 Margaret Wheatley (1992) *Leadership and the New Science: Learning about Organization from an Orderly Universe.* San Francisco, CA: Berrett-Koehler, p.149.
77 See Isabel M. Lyth (1989) *The Dynamics of the Social: Selected Essays.* London: Free Association Books, p.149.
78 See Gareth Morgan (1986) *Images of Organization.* Beverly Hills, CA: Sage Publications, pp.199–231.
79 Shirley P. Lowry (1982) *Familiar Mysteries: The Truth in Myth.* New York: Oxford University Press, p.131.

Procter & Gamble. That's how long it can take to forge new identities and relationships throughout all the levels of the organization.'[80]

APPLICATION TO HEALTHCARE

If it takes 25 years to change the culture of Procter & Gamble with approximately 130,000 employees, one can only imagine how long it would take to transform the culture of the NHS in Britain which employs about 1.5 million people. This comparison makes a mockery of policy documents regularly emanating from the NHS headquarters that assume cultural change can be easily achieved. The lesson is clear. Cultural change in healthcare, at any level, is always a slow process filled with uncertain outcomes. Radical organizational change requires long-term planning. Politicians in particular find this lesson extremely difficult to accept; they want changes quickly in order to please their constituents and become very annoyed when things do not move fast.[80]

Guideline 8: Since myths unconsciously shape feelings, thoughts and behaviours, it is easy for them to be manipulated in ways that blind people to reality, even exploit or oppress them[82]

When we speak of the 'culture unconscious', we simply mean that because symbols and myths are so much part of our inner selves, their existence and influence are apt to escape our conscious awareness. Social reality is so complex and ambiguous that insights that might threaten the security of our cultural myths are readily ignored or distorted in an effort to make it unambiguously simple. At best we are frequently controlled by our culture, and at worst oppressed. For example, Walter Wink speaks of the 'myth of redemptive violence'

---

80 Edgar H. Schein interviewed by D.L. Coutu (2002) 'The anxiety of learning.' *Harvard Business Review 80*, 3, 106. Procter & Gamble, a multinational manufacturer of a wide range of consumer goods, was listed in 2011 fifth in Fortune's Most Admired Companies. It is credited with many business innovations.

81 See Christopher Ham (2009) *Health Policy in Britain*. Basingstoke: Palgrave Macmillan, pp.316–317.

82 See Robert M. MacIver (1955) *The Web of Government*. London: Macmillan, p.4.

in Western society. He means it is taken for granted that violence is essential for a society's ongoing existence. Violence is offered as something that can solve conflicts. Even the threat alone of violence is able to prevent aggressors; the more power one has the more effective the threat.[83] Violence is redemptive in the sense that it returns society to a state of peace and justice. Television, cartoons, comic strips all reinforce this belief.[84] Psychologist Max Lerner, in a poignant passage written as Hitler was preparing for war, was extremely troubled by the obedient support evoked by the Führer. He prophetically cautioned that while the power of dictators comes from the 'symbols that they manipulate, the symbols depend in turn upon the entire range of associations that they evoke. The power of these symbols is enormous. Men [sic] possess thoughts, but symbols possess men.'[85]

Despite the extreme nature of these two examples, the lesson they contain is highly relevant to healthcare. The major focus of healthcare mythology remains unduly centred on hospitals, despite the urgency to improve public health and community care services for the mentally ill, disabled and elderly. For most people, the hospital has been made *the* symbol of health and it is difficult persuading them to the contrary. Try to close a local hospital and popular opposition will be immediate, vociferous and persistent, even though there are sound reasons for the closure. Governments and particular medical pressure groups have colluded in maintaining this mythological emphasis. Roy Griffiths, author of the British report *Community Care: An Agenda for Action*, wrote back in 1988: 'Community care has been talked of for thirty years and in few areas can the gap between the political rhetoric and policy on the one hand, and between policy and reality on the other, have been so great.'[86] Seven years later, Judith Allsop could report no change: 'The gap between rhetoric and reality is far from being closed and community care has entered a period of

83   Walter Wink (1992) *Engaging the Powers: Discernment and Resistance in a World of Domination.* Philadelphia, PA: Fortress, p.13.

84   Ibid., p.25; see also Peter Ackerman and Jack Duvall (2000) *A Force More Powerful: A Century of Nonviolent Conflict.* New York: Palgrave Macmillan, pp.457–459.

85   Max Lerner (1941) *The Ideas of the Ice Age.* New York: Viking Press, p.235.

86   Department of Health and Social Security (DHSS) (1988) *Community Care: An Agenda for Action* (Griffiths Report). London: HMSO, p.iv.

greater uncertainty and instability than hitherto.'[87] In 2012, British governments still, in essence, consider hospitals to be the primary focus of healthcare in their planning and they plan changes at the margin to allow for 'care in the community'.[88]

Technological creativity is deeply woven into our industrial mythology, and is no less a quality of healthcare. Medical technology saves lives and overcomes suffering, and is popular with the public, and very profitable for doctors and the health industry. But these costs are rising at increasingly unsustainable rates. Media interests, however, encouraged by industrial giants and some medical pressure groups, continually attempt to manipulate the mythology that if only more money could be given to advancing medical technology death itself could eventually be overcome. This campaign raises a key ethical issue, namely the clash between what medicine can do for the individual and what this will financially cost society as a whole. It is a struggle between individual rights and self-determination on the one hand, and the common good on the other.[89] All nations directly or indirectly must ration healthcare services simply because demands are infinite and resources are finite. The United States 'solves' the ethical dilemma by the capacity of individuals to pay; this means that low-income people simply cannot afford many medical services. The governments of Australia, New Zealand[90] and European countries including Britain ration by limitation of choice and placing people on waiting lists. In 1997 the British Medical Association (BMA) issued a draft revision of the Hippocratic Oath: 'I will use my training and professional standing to improve the community in which I work. I will treat patients equitably and support a fair and humane distribution of health resources...'.[91] It is not surprising, therefore,

---

87   Judith Allsop (1995) *Health Policy and the NHS: Towards 2000*. London: Longman, p.108.

88   See Iain Crinson (2009) *Health Policy: A Critical Perspective*. London: Sage Publications, p.174; Ian Greener (2009) *Healthcare in the UK: Understanding Continuity and Change*. Bristol: Policy Press, pp.29–30.

89   See Daniel Callahan (1998) *False Hopes: Why America's Quest for Perfect Health is a Recipe for Failure*. New York: Simon & Schuster, and (2009) *Taming the Beloved Beast: How Medical Technology Costs are Destroying Our Health Care System*. Princeton, NJ: Princeton University Press.

90   See John Butler (1999) *The Ethics of Health Care Rationing: Principles and Practices*. London: Cassell, pp.102–103.

91   British Medical Association (BMA) (1997) *BMA Annual Report of Council 1996–97*. London: BMA.

that the BMA has consistently campaigned in favour of the principle of equity in the NHS and against the inroads of the American-style healthcare system.[92]

Guideline 9: Myths contain polar opposites in an uneasy tension

One of the positive contributions of the anthropologist Claude Levi-Strauss to our understanding of mythology is his emphasis on their inherent polarities and the ability of myths to attempt to reconcile them.[93] For example, the founding myth of the United States contains several sets of polar opposites: the rights of the individual sovereign states over the rights of the federal government. Ideally these polar opposites must be kept in harmonious balance, but in practice one pole can dominate the other. Factions can form around both polar opposites in the mythology, as we see in the United States. Both factions claim they truly interpret the mythology. Then there is the polarity in healthcare mythology between hospital and community care, with the former being the dominant partner in the tension. And there are the polar tensions between medical clinicians and managers (explained in Chapter 3).

In the mythology of democracy, there are two complementary poles: the rights of the individual and those of the community. The third quality, 'fraternity', is the resulting balance between these two mythological poles. For North Americans, unlike Canadians, Australians, New Zealanders and the British, fraternity means that the rights of the individual are primarily to be respected, even though the common good may suffer. Hence, any attempt by the American government to redress the imbalance in favour of the common good is met with strong, highly organized emotional opposition. Healthcare reforms are branded, as we know in recent times, as 'socialized medicine', 'government-interference in private affairs', enough to destroy any effort to provide the much-needed healthcare to millions of people. Such is the power of mythology! Various other countries handle the tension between the opposing poles in healthcare mythology of 'universality' (public healthcare services)

92   See Pollock 2005, p.23.
93   See Edmund Leach (1970) *Levi-Strauss*. London: Fontana, pp.54–82.

and 'choice' (private healthcare) in different ways (see Figure 1.1). In Australia, for example, there is a hybrid system, with 40 per cent of hospitals in private hands; in Holland the mixed system allows for a significant degree of both universality and choice, while Canada, like Britain,[94] in 2012 emphasizes universality.[95]

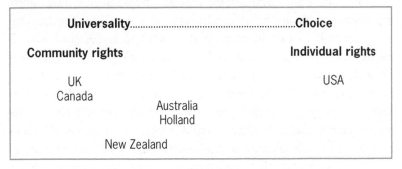

Figure 1.1: Healthcare systems[96]

Guideline 10: Individuals and cultures live and are revitalized through empathetic storytelling and listening

Myths are stories, as explained above, that give meaning to our lives in the past. The application of these myths to present realities is what is termed narrating or storytelling. In storytelling people apply myths from the past to what now concerns them in everyday life; in the process the myths are enlarged, changed or even put aside. Although Roland Barthes correctly describes human beings as 'narrating animals', because 'narrative is present in every age, in every place, in every society',[97] it is only since the 1980s that anthropologists have focused on the importance of narratives in all aspects of daily living, including people's experiences of sickness. Within a narrative, it is the plot that gives it a particular shape, that is, the plot gives meaning

---

94 Only 4 per cent of acute beds are provided by private companies in Britain. See 'Where lucre is still filthy: Squeamishness about profitmaking is hampering the government's bid to reform the public service.' (2011) *The Economist* (21 May), 60.

95 See Stewart 2009, pp.173–178.

96 For an overview of healthcare systems internationally, see George R. Palmer and Maria T. Ho (2008) *Health Economics: A Critical and Global Analysis*. Basingstoke: Palgrave Macmillan, pp.160–211.

97 Roland Barthes (1982) 'Introduction to the Structural Analysis of Narratives.' In Susan Sontag (ed.) *A Barthes Reader*. London: Cape, p.251.

to a series of events in a connecting and chronological sequence. In the words of the philosopher Paul Ricoeur: 'By plot I mean the intelligible whole that governs a succession of events in any story... A story is made out of events to the extent that plot makes events into a story.'[98]

The anthropological observations about storytelling have significant implications for healthcare. In storytelling the narrator is in control, so that listeners, if they wish to understand what is being said, must view reality from a different standpoint, even if they disagree with it. This requires of the listener the ability to empathize with the narrator, that is, storytelling calls the listener into a 'I–Thou' or 'heart-to-heart' relationship. By adhering to the biomedical model of healthcare (see Chapter 2), clinicians will focus too narrowly on biological phenomena and relate to patients as machines with parts that need repairing. They concentrate only on one aspect of a person's sickness. Patients, on the other hand, see their sickness in broader terms, a condition that affects their identity as a person with emotions, family and work obligations. They want to be listened to as people, not as broken-down machines in need of repair. Healthcare, in particular medicine, has rather slowly accepted the importance of narrative for relationship-centred diagnosis and healing. Many medical clinicians have been trained to cure the physical side of sickness, not to spend time for considering the inner illness of patients. The latter is the task of nurses, they would say. They are fearful of 'wasting time' by becoming involved in what patients are feeling. Yet this polarization of healthcare is dangerous, both for the medical people and patients.

Several authors describe that this relationship should be one of mutuality between clinicians and patients; a patient's human story should be influencing how the clinician views their own story and identity: 'When health care practitioners interact with patients, they jointly are writing new chapters or revising existing chapters in their stories – both the patients' and their own stories.'[99]

97   Paul Ricoeur (1980) 'Narrative time.' *Critical Inquiry* 7, 1, 171.
99   John D. Engel *et al.* (2008) *Narrative Health Care: Healing Patients, Practitioners, Profession, and Community.* Abingdon: Radcliffe Publishing, p.53.

EXAMPLE: PATIENT NARRATIVE

When I visit my doctor I tell him my story, the plot being my sickness and its symptoms; I go to him and not to a grocer because my cultural mythology assures me that doctors specialize in healing. I expect the doctor to listen. If not I feel dehumanized. In my story I identify myself at a particular time and place, that is, 'I am a sick person.' I no longer identify myself as a 'healthy person'. Sociologist Anthony Giddens describes this as the 'reflexive self', that is, a process whereby 'self-identity is constituted by the reflexive ordering of self-narratives'.[99] Oliver Sacks succinctly writes: 'It might be said that each of us constructs and lives a 'narrative,' and that this narrative *is* us, our identities.'[100] Implicit in my identification as a sick person is the mythologically-based assumption that my doctor will restore me to my normal self.

As for individuals, so also for organizational cultures. As will be explained more fully in Chapter 5, managers must be able to listen simultaneously to the stories of their organizations and of staff members. If the stories are interpreting the founding mythology of healthcare in vastly different ways, there is bound to be conflict, an overall organizational sickness.

Guideline 11: Culture profoundly influences the mental and physical health of patients *and* clinicians

There is an indisputable relationship between culture and people's health. For example, in Australia poverty is commonly viewed by people from an affluent culture as the victim's problem and not as a multifaceted cultural issue.[102] Likewise in the United States people who are poor, especially if they are single mothers, African Americans or Hispanics, are frequently stigmatized by members of

---

100 Anthony Giddens (1991) *Modernity and Self-Identity: Self and Society in the Late Modern Age.* Cambridge: Polity Press, p.244.
101 Oliver Sacks (1985) *The Man Who Mistook His Wife for a Hat and Other Clinical Tales.* New York: Summit Books, p.110.
102 See Alistair Grieg, Frank Lewins and Kevin White (2003) *Inequality in Australia.* Cambridge: Cambridge University Press, p.94.

the dominant culture. The impact of cultural factors on the health of the marginalized is ignored.[103] Clinicians, therefore, must be sensitive to the cultural factors that contribute to the problems, including poverty, of patients (see Chapter 2).[104]

Summary

○ Culture is the hidden language that influences how we feel, think and act; its constituent elements are symbols, myths and rituals. Symbols are felt meanings; myths are narrative symbols, that is, emotionally charged stories that articulate in imaginative ways basic values and truths for those who accept them; rituals are the visible expression of symbols and myths in actions. New myths are created and old ones maintained, constantly revised or lost completely because of a varied flow of forces, changing needs and new ways of seeing things.

○ There are three significant types of myths: public, operative and residual. The residual myth is one that has little or no impact on people's lives but which can become extremely influential in times of cultural turmoil.

○ Culture provides people with a sense of order and predictability in a world of threatening chaos; when people's expectations of order are significantly disrupted, there is fear and anxiety. The consequence is resistance.

○ Paradoxically, however, there can be no significant individual or organizational change unless there is an experience of cultural chaos, that is, the radical breakdown of order. Many projects incorporating change are never completed simply because the people involved cannot bear the phase of ambiguity or uncertainty that the chaos evokes. Since healthcare cultures and subcultures are under constant pressures from all sides to change as a result of technological innovations, changing needs of patients and financial restraints, it is inevitable that resistance to changes can be strong and sustained.

---

103 See Joel F. Handler and Yeheskel Hasenfield (2007) *Blame Welfare, Ignore Poverty and Inequality.* Cambridge: Cambridge University Press, pp.1–16.
104 See Malcolm MacLachlan (1997) *Culture and Health.* Chichester: John Wiley, pp.229–258; Pool and Geissler 2005, pp.117–140.

○ A culture is not homogeneous, but highly fragmented into a diversity of subcultures, such as are found in healthcare systems. Tensions between subcultures can be intense, especially when resources are limited and there are struggles over power.

○ If cultural change is to be positive in healthcare leaders need to be sensitive to the complexities and inherent resistances to cultural change.

Strategic implications
Policies

○ All healthcare systems, whether at state, regional or local levels, comprise many different cultures and subcultures.[105] Hence, it is essential that the correct understanding of culture is fundamentally important in devising, communicating and implementing healthcare reforms. Significant cultural changes demanded by reforms will take not days or months, but years of patient work, to be effective and respectful of the dignity of everyone involved. For this reason, training in the basic principles of social anthropology and related fields such as organizational behaviour is a necessary requirement in all management and employee development. Moreover, this training is especially important for certain roles such as policy-makers and those who must implement reforms, for example, administrators and clinicians.

○ Anthropological training must not be based on a didactic 'jug to mug' pedagogy. According to this pedagogy participants are likened to empty mugs waiting passively to be filled with the abstract theories of experts. If learning occurs, it is almost entirely at the intellectual level; people are not expected to examine their own emotional responses to what is handed down from above.

---

105 Sometimes the term 'multicultural' is used to describe the many different cultures and subcultures in healthcare systems, but this can be confusing. A multicultural system can be either 'demographic' or 'holistic'. The former simply means that the system contains different cultural groups; it says nothing about how they relate to one another. A holistic multicultural system, however, is one in which cultures maintain their identity but work together for the sake of the common good. *Ideally*, a healthcare system should be a holistic one.

○ Rather the inductive method needs to be adopted, that is, cultural training in healthcare institutions must begin with people's experiences – their fears, emotional reactions to events, their successes and failures. Only in this way can people begin to *feel* the power of culture in their own lives. Thus, inductive teaching aims to involve as many dimensions of the learner as is possible; its purpose is to foster integrated learning at the spiritual, cognitive, affective and behavioural levels, so that people are encouraged to make real attitudinal and behavioural changes. Inductive learning encourages critical thinkers in healthcare, people who are willing to critique the cultural world around them, as well as their own behaviour. It is a collaborative process involving 'all participants, teachers and learners alike, in a process of mutual vulnerability and risk taking, of personal challenge and learning'.[106]

Implementation

○ Skilled applied social anthropologists need to be appointed to departments of health to provide general strategic, humanizing advice and guidance for the cultural changes required by reforms.

○ Cultural sensitivity programmes, that is, programmes based on the inductive method, that foster in people an awareness of the power and complexity of culture in human relationships, need to be introduced into in-service programmes for all staff of healthcare systems; ongoing education will help to guarantee the welfare and safety not just of patients but also of staff members.

○ Since cultural changes in healthcare systems such as hospitals are more likely to succeed and be sustained if 'the why and wherefore of reform is taught in the undergraduate and early clinical training years',[107] cultural sensitivity programmes, based on the inductive method, need to be introduced at key points of students' training. Interdisciplinary teams cannot readily develop and be sustained without this integrated training.

---

106 Tony Hobbs (ed.) (1992) *Experiential Learning: Practical Guidelines.* London: Routledge, p.xiv.
107 Garling 2008b, p.5.

CHAPTER 2

Healthcare Models in Conflict

What about the Patient?

Is the physician, taken in that strict sense of which you are speaking, a healer of the sick or a maker of money?

(Plato)[1]

It's not the strongest species that survive, nor the most intelligent, but the ones most responsive to change.

(Charles Darwin)[2]

This chapter explains:

- that there are five models of healthcare: traditional, foundational, biomedical, social and economic rationalist

- that the Good Samaritan story is the residual myth of healthcare in the Western world; *inter alia* its key values are holistic health, equity and solidarity

- that the primary tension in healthcare is that between 'the mission' and 'the business'; in the economic rationalist model of healthcare the latter is dominant, contrary to the founding myth.

Healthcare facilities exist to serve patients. Yet this basic fact is often forgotten. Therefore governments and others find it necessary to remind people that healthcare facilities exist for the service of patients.

In 2005 the British government thought it necessary to recall the NHS to its primary focus, namely the welfare and safety of patients,

---

1   Plato, Book 1, 341c. In Robert M. Hutchins (ed.) (1952) *Great Books of the Western World, Plato 7.* Chicago, IL: William Benton, p.303.
2   Charles Darwin, quoted in *The Economist* (7 November 1999), 4.

not the well-being of clinicians and administrators![3] In 2008 officials in public hospitals in New South Wales, Australia, were urgently told, after reports of significant tragedies, that 'a new culture needs to take root which sees the patient's needs as the paramount central concern of the system and not the convenience of the clinicians and administrators'.[4] Donald Berwick of the Harvard Medical School and President Obama's appointee as Director of the Centers for Medicare and Medicaid Services, evoked widespread controversy in the United States when he reminded clinicians and others that patient-centred healthcare must be *the* priority in services. He wrote: 'I…believe that we…would be far better off if we professionals recalibrated our work such that we behaved with patients and families not as hosts in the care system, but as guests in their lives.'[5]

The purpose of this chapter is to refocus on the patient and to respond to questions such as: Why is the patient being forgotten? Should healthcare be subjected to the economic laws of supply and demand? Is it time to return healthcare to its original founding story of compassion, solidarity, equity and social justice?

Defining terms

The words 'disease', 'illness', 'sickness' and 'health' are constantly used indiscriminately of individuals or groups of people with rarely any clarification of what they mean. This failure is only adding to the difficulties and confusion in healthcare reforms.[6] *Disease* (including *injury*), if used scientifically or medically, describes breakdowns of a physiological and biological kind, whereas *illness*[7] connotes the inner or subjective experience of the individual who is aware that they have a disease.[8]

Indications of illness can be feelings of loneliness, helplessness, fears about the future, anger, even shame at times. The fact of being

3   See Department of Health 2005.
4   Garling 2008b, p.3. Robert Francis (Chariman) made similar comments in his inquiry into the Mid Staffordshire NHS Foundation Trust. See Francis 2010.
5   See Berwick 2009, p.559.
6   See David Seedhouse (1996) 'Theory or Practice?' In David Seedhouse (ed.) *Reforming Health Care: The Philosophy and Practice of International Health Reform.* Chichester: John Wiley, p.230.
7   See Cecil G. Helman (1994) *Culture, Health and Illness: An Introduction for Health Professionals.* Oxford: Butterworth, pp.101–145.
8   See Arthur Kleinman (1988) *The Illness Narratives: Suffering, Healing and the Human Condition.* New York: Basic Books, p.3; Pool and Geissler 2005, pp.52–75.

ill is the consequence of efforts on the part of the sick person and others to give some meaning to their experience. The distinction between disease and illness is of fundamental importance, so much so that we speak of *curing* a disease and *healing* the illness. Sometimes it is far more challenging to heal than to cure; the cure of disease can often be achieved through appropriate drugs or surgery, but the illness often requires the more difficult human skills of understanding and empathy. Finally, *sickness* is the attribution of ill health to a person by others, an ascription that may be made even when the person is not aware of illness, for example, in some forms of mental illness. Often the word *sickness* is used to mean both disease and illness, but this should not lessen the importance of distinguishing between them.[9]

There is increasing dissatisfaction with the limitations of scientific medicine (the biomedical model), particularly in disciplines like mental health, environmental studies and psychosocial aspects of public health interventions, for example, issues relating to drug and alcohol abuse, sexually transmitted diseases (STD), and human immunodeficiency virus (HIV). Scientific medicine is criticized for concentrating on disease, ignoring the reality of the inner pain of illness and the fact that the rightful functioning or harmony of the body is intimately related to psychological, cultural, environmental and spiritual factors. For example, to understand stress necessitates appreciation of the complex interplay between the body's immune system and such non-biological aspects as culture, social support and sense of self-worth.[10] Consequently there is a growing emphasis on a more holistic understanding of health which is regarded as synonymous with well-being, that is, a state characterized by contentment, prosperity and the fulfilment of fundamental human needs. According to the World Health Organization, therefore, health is 'a state of complete physical, mental and social well-being and not merely the absence of disease or infirmity'.[11] Health Canada has adopted a similarly expansive definition of health, seeing it as

> a state of social, mental, emotional, and physical well-being that is influenced by a broad range of factors, including biology and

---

9   See Bryan S. Turner (1995) *Medical Power and Social Knowledge,* 2nd edn. London: Sage Publications, pp.2–3.

10 See Richard Wilkinson and Michael Marmot (2003) *Social Determinants of Health: The Solid Facts,* 2nd edn. Geneva: World Health Organization.

11 World Health Organization WHO (1988) *Health Promotion Glossary.* Geneva: WHO, p.1.

genetics, personal health practices and coping skills, the social and physical environments, gender, socio-economic factors such as income and education, and cultural practices and norms.[12]

In addition to the active participation of individuals themselves, holistic healthcare involves not only medical professionals (many of whom are reluctant or find it difficult to accept this understanding of health) but also a wide range of agencies and disciplines. The task of governments is to develop a just society in and through which people can achieve harmonious well-being. Difficult political decisions must be made, such as resisting the excessive demands of the medical profession to have exclusive rights to determine public healthcare policies, and controlling economic rationalists who, in order to balance the books, would favour the rich to the disadvantage of people who are poor.

Healthcare: Models in conflict[13]

However, despite the growing acceptance of this more holistic appreciation of health governments and others pursue different healthcare policies and practices depending on their interpretation of the words 'health', 'disease', 'illness' and 'sickness'. Consequently, five different cultural models or types of healthcare can be identified: the traditional, foundational, biomedical, social and economic rationalist models.

Each model will be now explained and critiqued. An anthropological model aims to illumine complex reality by highlighting emphases and downplaying details or nuances. Nuanced explanations or details are omitted to allow us to grasp more clearly what is in fact a highly complex situation. Any particular culture is then compared with the model to see to what extent it resembles it or not. In a particular society or country it is possible for all the models to be simultaneously observable, with one model tending to be more influential than others. The models are not necessarily sequential, that is, it is not inevitable that the traditional model precedes the economic rationalist model.

---

12   Lorne Tepperman and Josh Curtis (2011) *Social Problems: A Canadian Perspective*, 3rd edn. Don Mills, Toronto: Oxford University Press, p.234.
13   See Arbuckle 2000, pp.3–94.

Traditional model

The traditional culture type is to be found very commonly among peoples in traditional Asia, Africa, parts of North, Middle and South America and the South Pacific. A person's identity cannot be separated from the identity of the group of their birth, such as the extended family, clan or tribe. Founding myths emphasize stability and tradition's sacredness, not change. The culture is a gift of the gods/ancestors and it cannot be questioned. The fear of being mocked by members of one's group or even punished by spirits if one transgresses traditional customs makes sure that there is conformity to the group's values and norms. Respect for patriarchal values is also a strong force in maintaining the healthy status quo. If women, in particular, break customs, then men, the protectors of tradition and stability, are deeply shamed. To avoid this happening and to maintain a sense of male honour, women must be kept in an inferior status and fully under men's control.

In traditional cultures mental, physical and social health are profoundly interrelated.[14] This model of health and healthcare is holistic in the sense that sickness is related to the whole person and the social and natural environments. Good health exists when people live in harmony with each other, their gods or spirits, and the environment. Thus sickness is not so much a biomedical condition as it is a social issue; it is primarily caused by social, not physical, factors. Even Hippocrates, a physician in the fourth century BCE, stressed holistic health when he insisted on the indivisible connection between a healthy mind and a healthy body. Likewise, Plato, in the same century:

> As you ought not to attempt to cure the eyes without the head, or the head without the body, so neither ought you to cure the body without the soul...for the part can never be well unless the whole is well and, therefore, if the head and body are well, you must begin by curing the soul.[15]

---

14 See Peter Morley (1978) 'Culture and the Cognitive World of Traditional Medical Beliefs: Some Preliminary Considerations.' In Peter Morley and Roy Wallis (eds) *Culture and Curing: Anthropological Perspectives on Traditional Medical Beliefs and Practices.* London: Peter Owen; Alice B. Child and Irvin L. Child (1993) *Religion and Magic in the Life of Traditional Peoples.* Englewood Cliffs, NJ: Prentice Hall, pp.129–139.

15 Plato, as cited by Gareth Tuckwell (1991) 'Christian health: A ministry to the whole person.' *Catholic Medical Quarterly 42,* 2, 13.

Health can be recovered through the use of a wide variety of folk medicines, but these are useless if social relationships and events are not renewed, and evil spirits ritually ejected, for it is they which are the primary cases of illness and sickness. Since sickness reflects the social circumstances of the individual it cannot be reduced to one physical cause such as a germ; rather, it is a form of evil that has complex social implications and causes. People accept that there are immediate and rational causes for misfortune, for example heart attacks can cause death. For every misfortune there is always a physical or natural cause. However, a further and far more important question, namely '*Why* is *this* person sick with cancer at *this* time and in *this* place?' or '*Why* did *this* person die with cancer?' must be answered in different ways. Often people believe that the ultimate cause of evil, in the form of sickness or death, is that ancestors punish the living for not showing them respect or for breaking tribal taboos. The living can also harm others through the intentional or unconscious use of magical forces, such as sorcery and witchcraft. Sorcery is the conscious use of magic to harm some person or group, whereas witchcraft is seen as a malign quality innate in a person. Witches, unlike sorcerers, are not necessarily conscious that they have this characteristic or are practising it. One day, when I was tramping through the bush in the Southern Highlands, Papua New Guinea, I came across a young man with a severe arm injury resting in a hut built far from the village. I offered to arrange for transport to a medical centre, but my suggestion was rejected by his father who commented:

> If we take him away he will surely die, because someone will work more sorcery on him. The government medical men can do nothing for him, unless we find out who has worked sorcery on him. It is surely a sorcerer who wants to harm him and our village because of something someone in our clan has done wrong.

His son's damaged arm, already dangerously infected, was due, he knew, to an accident, but its ultimate cause was surely due to someone working sorcery and wanting to inflict social disruption in the village. Unless the sorcerer could be discovered and the right magic used to counter the evil, the boy's arm would not heal and he would surely die. The father would not change his mind.

Examples of the traditional model

○ Among the aboriginal Yolngu community in Australia, when there is a death it is taken for granted that sorcery is the cause.[16]

○ The Azande people in Africa are very conscious that there are natural reasons for sickness, but they need additional explanations for sickness or misfortune. If a person enters the bush and is killed by an elephant, his relatives want to know why this happened. They acknowledge that the terrible mortal injuries caused death but they need to know why *this* man was killed by *this* elephant at *this* particular moment and in *this* specific place, and not someone else by other means and at another time and place. The answer is simple: he was the object of witchcraft or sorcery. Hence, for every occurrence of sickness or adversity there are two fundamental questions, namely *how* and *why* it happened; the second question is answered in terms of witchcraft or sorcery and the guilty person must be discovered and punished.[17]

○ In Melanesia, in the South Pacific, witchcraft and sorcery are believed to cause many types of sickness. For example, in Papua New Guinea the Tolai people assume that sorcery causes a headache and insanity.[18] Anthropologist Garry Trompf commented on urban life in Port Moresby, capital of Papua New Guinea: 'Certain deaths and instances of insanity among senior public servants…have even been attributed to sorcery by the broad consensus view of their national colleagues.'[19]

○ Maori people in New Zealand traditionally believed any failure of health was due to malignant spirits.[20] In contemporary times, when the cause of sickness is not easily understood or existing medical treatment is unsuccessful, Maoris often speak of *mate*

16 See Janice Reid (1983) *Sorcerers and Healing Spirits*. Sydney: Australian National University Press, p.152.
17 See Edward E. Evans-Pritchard (1937) *Witchcraft Oracles and Magic among the Azande*. Oxford: Clarendon Press.
18 See Garry W. Trompf (1994) *Payback: The Logic of Retribution in Melanesian Religions*. Cambridge: Cambridge University Press, pp.143–144.
19 Ibid., p.363.
20 See Peter Buck (1958) *The Coming of the Maori*. Wellington, NZ: Whitcombe and Tombs, pp.404–413.

ri (that is, 'Maori sickness'). The chief causes of *mate Maori*
ttributed especially to the breaking of sacred customs
and sorcery. Anthropologist Joan Metge wrote that the fear
'of sorcery is dormant most of the time, becoming dominant
only under stress in the face of the unaccountable. A diagnosis
of sorcery usually involves attributing responsibility to some
particular person…known to envy or have been offended
by the victim.'[21] Once sorcery is diagnosed and neutralized,
'sorcery recoils on the originator',[22] whose sickness or death is
considered to prove guilt.

In Samoan society, noted Ineke Lazar, culture-bound disorders
(*ma'i aitu*) included a severe form of hysterical psychosis, other
neurotic symptoms and certain physiological conditions. A
common complaint, she found, in the Los Angeles Samoan
community is that, in the words of her informants, 'Samoan
illnesses do not show up on X-rays. So, the doctor does not
know what to do.' The people turn to traditional Samoan
therapists specializing in *aitu* ('spirit')-related illnesses, who use
what they believe is spirit medicine. They must find out where
the spirit comes from and why it is troubling the living.[23] For
example, it was reported in 1971 that in a contemporary Samoan
village a man had become deranged and was considered to be
possessed by an *aitu*. A family member acknowledged that he
had not properly cared for his aunt when she was alive. The
extended family met and concluded that her *aitu* was punishing
them. They then pushed a pipe into her grave and filled it with
boiling water and the man was restored to good health.[24]

Four main functions are achieved through traditional healing rituals
in these pre-modern cultures. The rituals are *diagnostic*, to discover
not only the cause of the sickness, but also *who* is causing it; *curative*,
that is, they aim to heal the person and restore order and harmony
once more to the community; *preventive*, to protect people from

---

21   Joan Metge (1976) *The Maoris of New Zealand*. London: Routledge & Kegan Paul, p.92.
22   Ibid.
23   See Ineke M. Lazar (1985) '*Ma'I Aitu*: Culture-bound illnesses in a Samoan migrant
      community.' *Oceania 55*, 3, 161–181.
24   See Richard A. Goodman (1971) 'Some *Aitu* beliefs of modern Samoans.' *Journal of the
      Polynesian Society 80*, 4, 463–479.

attacks of evil spirits or sorcerers; and *causative*, that is, magical rites to ensure that things are to one's advantage.[25]

In traditional cultures there are a variety of specialists, such as oracles, shamans or diviners, and methods to discern precisely which spirit or person is causing the evil, the reasons why and the necessary remedies. Among the African Azande, for example, oracles discover if witchcraft is likely to interfere with a particular task and identify the witches responsible for problems. In the termite oracle, for example, two sticks are placed in a termite mound for a day; the answer is found by noting which stick was eaten first. The termite oracle is considered to be less reliable than the intricate and costly poison oracle which needs to be used to tackle the identified witch and to begin the vengeance process when death is involved.[26] Shamanism is a term for an intricate mixture of religious and ethno-medical beliefs and practices found among cultures in Asia, Africa and aboriginal America. It claims, as does witchcraft, the use of spiritual powers to counter the influence of enemies and cause or cure disease. While sickness may have several causes, the most important is due to the loss of the soul through evil forces. The shaman's skill, exercised through a trancelike state, is to find the missing soul in some hidden section of the cosmic world and restore it to the sick person.[27]

Foundational model

The philosopher Charles Taylor, when reflecting on the origins of Western civilization, concludes that the story of the Good Samaritan 'can be seen as one of the original building blocks out of which our modern universalist moral consciousness has been built'.[28] Social ethicist Chris Marshall, of Victoria University, New Zealand, wrote that the story 'carries tremendous rhetorical power, for it evokes one of the most seminal narratives in the Western cultural tradition'. He continued: 'Indeed, it is hard to think of another story that has

---

25 For analyses of witch doctors and health see E. Fuller Torrey (1972) *Witchdoctors and Psychiatrists: The Common Roots of Psychology and Its Future*. New York: Harper & Row; Susan Fernando (1991) *Mental Health, Race and Culture*. London: Macmillan, pp.150, 166.

26 See Lucy Mair (1969) *Witchcraft*. New York: McGraw Hill, pp.76–101.

27 See Arthur Kleinman (1980) *Patients and Healers in the Context of Culture: An Exploration of the Borderland between Anthropology, Medicine, and Psychiatry*. Berkeley, CA: University of California Press, pp.203–258.

28 Charles Taylor (2007) *The Secular Age*. Cambridge: Cambridge University Press, p.738.

been more influential in moulding personal and political virtue... It is a story that still serves, even in contemporary secular society, as a useful reference point for measuring policy options.'[29] Testimony to the story's noteworthy legacy is simply the continuing general use in society of the phrase 'Good Samaritan' as an example of self-sacrificing concern for others.[30] In the early centuries of the Christian era, the story (technically called a *parable*) became the public and operative founding myth among Christians in general, and later the monasteries in particular, obliging them to care for the sick in whom body and soul are united. Every stranger in need is a neighbour, the image of God, to whom the love of God ought to be demonstrated. Subsequently, 'permanent charitable institutions sprang up within a generation or two after the end of the persecution of the Christians' in the fourth century.[31] Christians formed 'a miniature welfare state in an empire which for the most part lacked social services'.[32] At the heart of this founding healthcare myth are the values of solidarity, equity, compassion, mercy and social justice.

Therefore, it was not surprising that Barbara Castle, when Secretary of State for Health in Britain in the 1970s and a close colleague of Aneurin Bevan, founder of the NHS, stated that the NHS 'is the nearest thing to the embodiment of the Good Samaritan that we have in any aspect of our public policy'.[33] In this statement, Castle correctly identified the Good Samaritan story as the ultimate founding myth of healthcare throughout the Western world, with its emphasis in modern times on good quality healthcare, as a fundamental human right, rooted in human relationships and trust between health workers and patients. To ignore this human right is an act of violence, an affront to the dignity of the person.

29   Chris Marshall (2011) '"Go and Do Likewise": The Parable of the Good Samaritan and the Challenge of Public Ethics.' In Jonathan Boston, Andrew Bradstock and David Eng (eds) *Ethics and Public Policy: Contemporary Issues.* Wellington, NZ: Victoria University Press, p.53.
30   Ibid.; C. Daniel Batson (1975) 'Attribution as a mediator of bias in helping.' *Journal of Personality and Social Psychology 32*, 3, 455–466; Hanokh Dagan (1999) 'In defense of the Good Samaritan.' *Michigan Law Review 97*, 5, 1115–1200. Martin Luther King, Jr, reflecting on the Good Samaritan story, insisted that the lesson is not just about charity, but it must be accompanied by structural and systemic transformation based on justice. See Marshall 2011, p.53.
31   Gary B. Ferngren (2009) *Medicine and Health Care in Early Christianity.* Baltimore, MD: Johns Hopkins University Press, p.145.
32   Paul Johnson, cited by Ferngren, ibid., p.138.
33   Barbara Castle, cited by Klein 2006, p.86.

The stories of the formation of the welfare state, therefore, in countries like Britain, New Zealand, Australia and Canada[34] would have been deeply influenced by the residual myth of the Good Samaritan. The social democratic founders may not have been conscious of this, but they certainly drew on the values inherent in the myth, such as solidarity, equity, compassion and justice. Just as the wounded Jew in the parable had a right to receive the care from the Samaritan, so also everyone today has the right to healthcare. It is not a commodity to be bought only by those who can afford it. Aneurin Bevan often emphasized this fundamental right:

> Society becomes more wholesome, more serene and spiritually healthier, if it knows that its citizens have at the back of their consciousness the knowledge that not only themselves, but all their fellows have access, when ill, to the best that medical skill can provide.[35]

In 1946 he had even more forcefully declared that 'it is repugnant to a civilized community for hospitals to have to rely upon charity'.[36] Michael Savage (1872–1940), the New Zealand Prime Minister from 1935 to 1940 and the founder of the nation's welfare state, was of the same mind: 'I want to see that people have security... I want to see humanity secure against poverty, secure in illness in old age...What is more valuable in our Christianity than to be our brother's keepers in reality.'[37] Savage also called the Social Security Act 1938 'applied Christianity'.[38] There is no denying the explicit and implicit influence of Christian thinking on the original formation of the philosophy of the welfare state. Sections of the Church of England contributed significantly to the final shape of the welfare state in Britain, most notably through the influence of William Temple, Archbishop of Canterbury, particularly through his

---

34 Tommy Douglas (1904–1986), architect of universal healthcare in Canada, was deeply influenced by the Social Gospel movement, which combined Christian principles with social reform.
35 Aneurin Bevan, cited by Margaret Whitehead (1993) 'Is it Fair? Evaluating the Equity Implications of the NHS Reforms.' In Ray Robinson and Julian Le Grand (eds) *Evaluating the NHS Reforms*. London: King's Fund, p.210.
36 Aneurin Bevan, quoted by A. O'Hagan (2011) *London Review of Books* (3 March), 34.
37 Michael Savage, cited by the Department of Social Security (1950) *The Growth and Development of Social Security in New Zealand*. Wellington, NZ: Government Printer, 17.
38 Ibid.

best-selling book *Christianity and Social Order* (1942). Temple created the expression 'welfare state' in opposition to the 'power state'.[39]

Good Samaritan story: Residual founding myth

To grasp the relevance and the power of the Good Samaritan parable or story, we first need to appreciate the general cultural environment at the time it was told. Only by returning to the cultural background of the story is it possible to grasp its extraordinary richness. Without this cultural approach, the parable will remain so domesticated in the popular imagination that its extensive relevance and the reason that people like Barbara Castle and others found it so helpful can be missed.

The story is a myth in the sense used in Chapter 1 and should be analysed from a social anthropological perspective. Like all myths, this one is far more complicated than it may seem to the general reader. In the Hebrew culture of the time, in which few could read or write, parables were a common and picturesque form of communication. They were fictitious stories that conveyed critically important messages. And like all myths they were structured to engage the imagination of listeners, frequently with a humorous or incongruous ending to them. The unexpected usually occurs with a rather stunning action by one of the leading characters or an unanticipated change of events; the apparent ordinariness of the parable is transformed by this surprising twist. While parables were fictitious stories, nonetheless they were always about situations and characters that people would recognize. Such was the case with the Good Samaritan parable.

Five pivotal people were involved: the victim, the Samaritan as caregiver, the priest, the Levite, who was a lawyer, and the innkeeper. The Levite belonged to an order of cultic officials, inferior to the priests but nonetheless a privileged group in Jewish society. The story on the surface is simple enough. A traveller is gravely injured by bandits and left to die on the roadside. Two esteemed pillars of society, namely the priest and lawyer, refuse to go to his aid. However, one despised by the Jewish people – a Samaritan – responds immediately to the victim's plight. To appreciate the quality of the

---

39   See Francis Davis, Elizabeth Paulhus and Andrew Bradstock (2008) *Moral, but No Compass: Government, Church and the Future of the Welfare State.* Chelmsford: Mathew James, p.29.

Samaritan's actions it is helpful to focus the story around fi
of violence: physical, social, ritual, racial and occupational.

VIOLENCE

The first act of violence is physical, namely, the assault by bandits
of an innocent man. At the time it was common for gangs of thugs
to terrorize wealthy travellers, rob them and often give the proceeds
to the poor.[40] The second act of violence is ritual. Because there
is blood on the victim he is automatically stigmatized as impure,
untouchable and therefore a social outcast. Being branded as defiled
would have caused intense inner pain. People would hesitate to help
him because that would render them ritually impure, necessitating
lengthy ceremonies of purification. He is also stripped naked. This
is the third act of violence.[41] To strip a person naked in public is the
ultimate act of subjugation and social marginalization. Therefore, in
describing the victim's plight, the storyteller is first concentrating
on the illness aspect, that is, the victim's interior suffering – the
shame, loneliness, marginalization. This illness quality is far more
excruciatingly painful for the victim than the actual physical suffering.

The priest and Levite, two pillars of Jewish culture, represent
religious fundamentalism of their times. The Hebrew cultural
tradition required that people must show compassion, especially to
people who were poor and marginalized, but Jewish fundamentalists
discarded this obligation, developing instead a religion that focused
on external conformity to rituals of accidental importance. The priest
returning from the Temple in Jerusalem to his home in the country
refused to help for two reasons: he feared being attacked by bandits
if he delayed, but, more importantly, he was not prepared to be
defiled by touching the victim.

The figure of the Samaritan traveller highlights a fourth form
of violence. Jews regarded the heretical Samaritans as religiously
and racially inferior and the Samaritans had similar views of
their Jewish neighbours. The story contains yet a fifth example of
violence: occupational prejudice and discrimination. Traders in oil

---

40   See Bruce J. Malina and Richard L. Rohrbaugh (1992) *Social-Science Commentary on the Synoptic Gospels*. Minneapolis, MN: Fortress Press, p.404.
41   John J. Pilch and Bruce J. Malina (eds) (1993) *Biblical Social Values and their Meaning*. Peabody, MA: Hendrickson, p.121.

and wine, like the Samaritan, were stigmatized because both Jews and Samaritans considered oil and wine sellers as very shady people indeed, even criminals. For this reason, those who listened to the storyteller would have been not just surprised, but shocked to hear that such a person – one marginalized by Jewish culture – became the caregiver. The Samaritan, like the victim, knew the pain of social rejection and loneliness. So, the surprising twist to the story. Though there were two strikes stigmatizing him, it was this Samaritan – one considered to be religiously and racially inferior, as well as occupationally questionable – who became the caregiver. In brief, the Samaritan was socially and racially a disabled person. Yet he was the one who spontaneously acted to help the victim.

There is another unexpected aspect to the involvement of the fifth character in the story, the innkeeper. The inn in the story was a den of thieves, and the head thief was the innkeeper, yet he was prepared to help the victim, for a price. The Samaritan sought to build relationships with this shady character, but the caregiver was no dreamer, out-of-touch with the weaknesses of human nature. Knowing what to expect from the innkeeper, the Samaritan simply bribed him in order to guarantee that the patient would be looked after and kept alive. He left the innkeeper a certain amount, but promised more when he returned.[42]

The story details the qualities of the Samaritan. He was courageous because he risked his own life by getting off his horse, his only form of protection, becoming in consequence vulnerable to attack by bandits. Every moment he was off the horse the physical danger to himself intensified. His courage was further tested when he walked the horse to avoid exacerbating the sufferings of the victim, thus further risking an attack. The listeners to the story know that the road from Jericho to Jerusalem, with its tortuous bends and rocky sides, is ideal for robbers.

In addition to the physical risks there were the ritual and social costs of touching the victim. We were told that the caregiver bandaged his wounds, pouring oil and wine on them. In order to bandage the victim, the Samaritan must touch him, but since the Samaritans had similar laws about ritual impurity, the caregiver himself became ritually unclean. This willingness to go to the margins of society in

---

See Malina and Rohrbaugh 1992, pp.346–348.

his ministry of healing defined the depth of his compassion. The victim would have been deeply comforted by this touch. At last there was someone who felt with him in his anguish of ritual and social marginalization. Never in the story are we told that the victim physically survives, but through the Samaritan's touch we know with certainty that the victim's inner pain was healed.

The Samaritan exercised the gift of hospitality. He gave of his substance or capital – the oil and wine – which he had intended to sell at the market. In biblical cultures hospitality is never restricted to entertaining one's friends or family members, but primarily refers to receiving strangers and a willingness to share one's capital goods with them without the expectation of return. Outsiders are invited to cease being strangers and become instead honoured guests.[43] Jewish law requires this because, as the Israelites had been strangers in Egypt, so they should themselves show hospitality to strangers. The ancient Book of Leviticus says: 'You will treat resident aliens as though they were native-born and love them as yourself' (Lev 19:34). Jesus would develop this further, not just in this parable, but through his example and his teachings. People who would receive the disciples of Jesus would, in fact, be receiving Jesus himself. To offer or refuse hospitality meant that the Gospel had been accepted or rejected.[44]

In summary, the dramatic paradox of the story, that would have shocked contemporary listeners, is that a Samaritan, one considered a religious heretic, a culturally and occupationally inferior person, spontaneously aided the dying man. Through his actions the Samaritan broke through the many layers of violence. Those in power who should act, the priest and the lawyer, turned their backs on the injured and marginalized victim. The relevance of the story down through the centuries is strikingly evident in the values contained within it.

43   See Pilch and Malina 1993, pp.104–107.
44   See A.J. Malherbe (1993) 'Hospitality.' In Bruce M. Metzger and Michael D. Coogan (eds) *The Oxford Companion to the Bible.* New York: Oxford University Press, pp.292–293; Brendan Byrne (2000) *The Hospitality of God: A Reading of Luke's Gospel.* Sydney: St Pauls Publications, pp.100–102.

VALUES

Values are of two kinds: *final*, that is, meaning a desired end state, and those termed *instrumental*, that is, those actions that are adequate or essential to achieve the desired end.[45] Final values in the story are: holistic health (the illness and disease are treated), equity (care is given with no reference to payment) and solidarity/social justice (peace and justice are restored as all peoples have fundamental rights to security and good health). Instrumental values are: respect for human dignity; compassion/empathy (the caregiver identifies with the feelings of the victim); hospitality (the caregiver shares his own capital wealth – oil, wine and money – with the victim); courage; dialogue (the caregiver's relationship with the innkeeper); and efficiency (the caregiver skilfully uses his talents and capital goods in the service of the victim).

The fundamental binary opposition (see Chapter 1) in the mythology of the Good Samaritan is that between what I call 'the mission' and 'the business'.[46] The former, the mission, is to be the driving force behind the latter (Figure 2.1). The mission pole contains the values that are to guide all caregivers: compassion, empathy, communitarian solidarity, a preference for the marginalized and social justice. The Samaritan is sensitive to the distinction between disease and illness. While he does not neglect the disease or injury aspect, his primary concern is with the illness, the inner pain of the victim. Hence, his emphasis on compassion, human solidarity and social inclusion; by his actions the Samaritan overcomes the five forms of violence. By touching the victim, the Samaritan caregiver expressed solidarity and compassion for the victim, for he was himself ritually marginalized by this action. His willingness to move to the margins of society as a caregiver demonstrates the depth of his compassion. The victim was deeply comforted by this touch. At last, there was someone who felt with him in his anguish and marginalization by the priest and Levite. The Samaritan was also immensely courageous. He constantly risked his life on the bandit-ridden road for the sake of the victim.

45   See Dolan *et al.* 2006, pp.32–33.
46   See Brad H. Young (1998) *The Parables: Jewish Tradition and Christian Interpretation.* Peabody, MA: Hendrickson, pp.101–188.

The Mission driving..The Business

Final values
Holistic health
Equity
Solidarity/social justice

Instrumental values
Respect
Compassion/empathy
Hospitality
Courage
Dialogue
Efficiency

Figure 2.1: Foundational model of healthcare

But there are less obvious 'business' dimensions to the parable. The Samaritan was a shrewd business man. If he had not been an efficient wine and oil merchant he would have had no material goods of wine, oil and money to assist the victim. His management skills are further evident in the way he related to the innkeeper. At the time the parable was told innkeepers were considered to be thieves, out to rob and kill unwary travellers. So, the alert Samaritan wisely bribed the innkeeper in order to care for the victim. An example of the values of efficiency and excellence!

There is an obvious convergence between these values inherent in the Good Samaritan story and the founding values of the welfare states in such countries as Britain, the member states of the European Union (EU), New Zealand, Australia and Canada. For example, when the tax-funded NHS was created in Britain in the late 1940s the emphasis was on the values of comprehensiveness, healthcare to cover all health needs; universalism, health services to be the same everywhere, including the poorest parts of the country; and solidarity and equitable access to health services based on need, not the ability to pay. In the EU, it was decided, in 2006, that the core values should be: universality, access to good quality healthcare for every person living in the EU; equitable access to healthcare regardless of ethnicity, gender, age, social status and ability to pay; and solidarity, people's fundamental right to healthcare and the obligation of governments to ensure that this right is financially respected.[47] Implicit in the formation of these healthcare systems are the other values at the heart of the Good Samaritan story, such as respect, compassion and dialogue.

Biomedical model

This model of healthcare is especially popular in Western societies. Ill health is regarded as a quality of the body, or more particularly, the inability of the body, for whatever reason, to function to its optimal level. In this model, the body is likened to a machine and disease is a breakdown of this machine. The inner affliction, or *illness* quality of sickness, is of no concern, that is, the state of the patient's mind is unimportant in medical diagnosis and treatment. Two factors alone are important: the *disease* and the *engineering* of the body back to health. Disease is a biological abnormality in a particular part of the body; the emphasis is now less on the symptoms supplied by the patient, as is the case in the previous two models, and more on signs that can theoretically be scientifically calculated, often with the use of instruments, by a medical expert, whose role is to engineer the body back to good health again through medical technology that is grounded in exact scientific laboratory procedures. Health, according to this model, is a commodity. It is a commodity that people possess and, if it is lost, it can be returned by medical engineering. As with any commodity, investors can take out insurance to cover loss or harm.

This model of healthcare evolved as a consequence of the dramatic development of scientific knowledge about the causes of disease, the rapid establishment of teaching hospitals and medical institutes committed to the study of the human body. Its historical and philosophical roots are to be found in the sixteenth century, reinforced by the writings of the Enlightenment, and in the nineteenth century, when the pivotal concept of modern culture became the *self*, not the group. The pre-eminent position of the person and the belief that human progress is inexorable found support in the development of classical physics. Matter was thought to be the foundation of all life and the material world was assumed to be an

---

47   See Scott L. Greer (2009) *The Politics of European Union Health Policies*. Maidenhead: Open University Press, p.7.

orderly machine consisting of elementary parts. In general, scientists and Western society adopted these assumptions of classical physics, deeply affecting the thinking of politicians, social commentators, economists, philosophers and the emerging medical profession.

René Descartes

Influential in the development of this model was the French philosopher and scientist René Descartes (1596–1650); his insights had a profound impact mainly because of the implications of his famous axiom 'I think, therefore I am.' In light of this saying, it was concluded that individuals must equate their identity with their rational mind. The idea of an integrated body, mind and spirit no longer made any sense. This encouraged people to ignore their bodies as avenues of knowing and, unlike in the previous model, to separate themselves from their surrounding natural environment. Given his emphasis on rationality, forms of knowledge that do not conform to norms of precise thinking were not considered to be valuable. Hence, knowledge through symbols and myths had no validity. In other words, feelings do not provide any valid insight into reality and, consequently, into the health of individuals.

Isaac Newton

The second influential figure was Sir Isaac Newton (1642–1727), mathematician and theoretical and experimental physicist, who claimed that the universe acted like a logical and materially structured machine with smoothly interchangeable parts that result in regulated order. These assumptions supported the view that the human body also operated like a machine. And as living organisms were thought to be machines built from parts, so also were cultures. The latter could be divided up and sections destroyed without any guilt because of this mechanistic view. Such a view supported ruthless colonialism, extreme capitalism and eventually the rise of Social Darwinism. The latter assumes that societies evolve through natural conflicts between social groups. The best adapted and most successful social groups survive these conflicts, raising the evolutionary levels of society. Government intervention, in healthcare, for example, wrongfully interferes with this dynamic.

While the benefits of the biomedical model are not denied, when the model is over-emphasized it has distinct disadvantages. First, it has led to an excessive concentration on acute hospital services to the detriment of primacy care facilities. Resources are focused on patients who are attractive from a technical point of view, while those with disabilities, older people and those with mental ill health are often left to survive in inappropriate conditions.[48]

Second, the biomedical model has become the dominant model of healthcare, both as regards its overall acceptability by the medical profession and the general public, and in terms of government funding priorities.[49] Until recently doctors long held the monopoly in determining the allocation of resources in healthcare, reinforcing the central role of the biomedical model of healthcare. In 1934 the American Medical Association declared its policy: 'All features of medical service...should be under the control of the medical profession. No other body or individual is legally or educationally equipped to exercise such control.'[50] The medical lobby has been particularly vociferous whenever governments have sought to establish welfare and healthcare services. For example, under the Social Security Act of 1938, the New Zealand government intended general practitioner, hospital, pharmaceutical and maternity services to be free and universal. The first of these plans created significant and long-lasting hostility between the medical profession and the government.[51] Exactly the same reactions have occurred in Britain, Canada and Australia. The British Medical Association compelled Aneurin Bevan to weaken aspects of the NHS before its introduction in 1948. Likewise, in the United States, where any effort by the federal government to reform the health system has evoked strong opposition from the medical profession whenever the private practice of medicine has been threatened.

---

48 See Pollock 2005, p.77.
49 See James Knight (1998) 'Models of Health.' In John Germov (ed.) *Second Opinion: An Introduction to Health Sociology.* Oxford: Oxford University Press, p.153.
50 American Medical Association, cited by Edward Rayack (1978) *Professional Power and American Medicine: The Economics of the American Medical Association.* New York: World Publishing, p.9.
51 See Derek A. Dow (1995) *Safeguarding the Public Health: A History of the New Zealand Department of Health.* Wellington, NZ: Victoria University Press, p.122.

Critique

This medical dominance has been severely critiqued by observers like Michel Foucault,[52] Ivan Illich and, to a lesser extent, by sociologist Talcott Parsons. In the 1950s Parsons critiqued the model to the degree that he reaffirmed the central importance of the 'total human individual'.[53] He asserted that sickness must be assessed not only in biological and economic ways, but also according to people's psychological and social aspects. But he held to the dangerous assumption that the doctor is selfless and objective and that patients should be passive, compliant and grateful to the doctor because the doctor has the superior knowledge. This gives the medical profession power to apply to people diagnostic labels that have serious moral, social and individual consequences.[54] This can happen, claims Graham Scambler, most knowingly when the situations being diagnosed are personally or socially stigmatizing. Stigmatizing conditions can be defined as conditions 'that set their possessors apart from "normal" people, that mark them as socially unacceptable or inferior beings'.[55]

Foucault (see Chapter 1), aiming to trace the historical development of medical interest in the human body, claims that the 'body is the ultimate site of political and ideological control...and regulation',[56] and modern medicine has developed considerable power in society through a process of 'clinical gaze' or surveillance of the human body labelling it as 'deviant or normal, hygienic or unhygienic, as controlled or needful of control'.[57] For example, people who have mental ill health or learning disabilities have often been branded as deviant and consequently marginalized from society. In the 1980s AIDS/HIV patients suffered this fate.

Illich's radical thesis is that development has become an addiction to need, not liberation from scarcity. When this is applied to healthcare

---

52 See Michel Foucault (1965) *Madness and Civilization: The History of Insanity in the Age of Reason*. New York: Random House and (1975) *The Birth of the Clinic: An Archaeology of Medical Perception*. New York: Vintage Books.
53 Talcott Parsons (1970) *The Social System*. London: Routledge & Kegan Paul, p.431.
54 See Margaret Stacey (1988) *The Sociology of Health and Healing*. London: Routledge, pp.160–176.
55 Graham Scambler (1997) 'Deviance, Sick Role and Stigma.' In Graham Scambler (ed.) *Sociology as Applied to Medicine*, 4th edn. London: W.B. Saunders, p.173.
56 Deborah Lupton (1994) *Medicine as Culture: Illness, Disease and the Body in Western Societies*. London: Sage Publications, p.23.
57 Ibid.

services, this means that the primary purpose of the medical profession is to serve its own social status and financial needs rather than the needs of patients. His book opens with this disquieting statement: 'The medical profession has become a major threat to health. The disabling impact of professional control over medicine has reached the proportions of an epidemic.'[58] This epidemic he terms 'iatrogenesis', that is, the encouraging of a professional mystique that conceals the fact that doctors are partly the reason for a large amount of the sickness which they claim to cure. For Illich, 'clinical iatrogenesis' is the false diagnosis resulting in sickness, even death; 'social iatrogenesis', means that the doctors' dominance over our bodies is so great that our own bodies become as if they were foreign to us, for example, the natural act of childbirth has become a medical process. Finally, here is 'cultural iatrogenesis', that is, doctors have made the natural experiences of pain and death prohibited topics for others. By encouraging us to deny these experiences doctors make it increasingly difficult for us to live fully and naturally. In dramatic terms he writes that excessive power of the medical profession has even ended the process of 'natural death'. 'Western man [sic] has lost', he asserts, 'the right to preside at his act of dying. Health, or the autonomous power to cope, has been expropriated down to the last breath.'[59]

The feminist critique of the medicalization of healthcare can also be scathing. For a long time now women have become subject to the advice and control of the medical profession as to when and how they are to give birth; the process has been transformed from a natural into a medical event.[60] Again, women are more likely to be typed as suffering from clinical depression than men, but the oppressive cultural factors to which women are often subject are rarely identified as important. Describing the British situation, a review in the mid-1990s stated that women as patients 'suffer rather than benefit from views which presume their physical

---

58   Ivan Illich (1990) *Limits to Medicine: Medical Nemesis – The Expropriations of Health*. London: Penguin, p.11.
59   Ibid., p.210.
60   See Elaine Papps and Mark Olssen (1997) *Doctoring Childbirth and Regulating Midwifery in New Zealand: A Foucauldian Perspective*. Palmerston North, NZ: Dunmore, pp.55–81. Following the insights of Foucault, the authors trace the process of medicalization of childbirth in New Zealand from the turn of the century to the passing of the Nurses Amendment Act in 1990, which restored the right of midwives to take sole charge in birth situations and gave them the right to prescribe drugs.

and/or psychological weakness...The sexual stereotypes of women as potentially sick...and emotionally unstable have militated against a rational approach to women's illnesses.'[61]

Paulo Freire's critique of education systems in general can also be directed at the educational system that developed around the biomedical model. He critiques pedagogical systems that reinforce unjust structures in society. He condemns systems that suffer from 'narration sickness', that is, where all the power rests with teachers; students must submissively, without question, accept the information given from above. He calls for 'conscientization', that is, a process whereby people become aware of, and question, this oppressive process.[62] This method has application to health education at two levels. Junior doctors are to be encouraged to question educational systems that deny them an active voice in their training. Moreover, people also have the right to insist that, as patients, they are not to remain passive in the presence of members of the medical profession.[63]

A final weakness of this model is that it reduces attention to the socioeconomic and environmental causes of disease. It ignores other findings, as expressed by Professor David Locker, University of Toronto: 'The main conclusion...is that patterns of health and disease are largely the product of social and environmental influences. Although health and illness may involve biological agents and processes, they are inseparable from the social settings in which people live.'[64]

In summary, the biomedical model rests firmly within 'the business' side of the founding myth of healthcare, thus distorting the original emphasis on the myth's mission pole. It is primarily about the cure of the individual's physical body and scientifically measurable results, not about the health of the full person or the socioeconomic injustices that cause disease. It ignores the relationship between biological processes and the unjust environments in which people live and work, such as dangerous work locations, poor housing and unemployment.

---

61   Sheila Hillier and Graham Scambler (1997) 'Women as Patients and Providers.' In Graham Scambler (ed.) *Sociology as Applied to Medicine*, 4th edn. London: W.B. Saunders, p.30.

62   See Paulo Freire (1972) *Pedagogy of the Oppressed*. Harmondswoth: Penguin, pp.45, 47.

63   See John J. Macdonald (1992) *Primary Health Care: Medicine in Its Place*. London: Earthscan, pp.158–161; Nina Wallerstein (1997) 'Freirian Praxis in Health Education and Community Organizing.' In Meredith Minkler (ed.) *Community Organizing and Community for Health*. New Brunswick, NJ: Rutgers University Press, pp.195–211.

64   David Locker (1997) 'Social Causes of Diseases.' In Graham Scambler (ed.) *Sociology as Applied to Medicine*, 4th edn. London: W.B. Saunders, p.30.

Social model

The next model, the social model, focuses particularly on the prevention of sickness. It does not deny that pathological or individual psychological factors cause sickness. However, it assumes that health and sickness cannot be fully understood or addressed unless the cultural and economic causes of poverty, unemployment, pollution, inappropriate personal and community lifestyles, class and gender prejudice are tackled. As the Marmot Review recently stated: 'Inequalities in health arise because of inequalities in society... In England, people living in the poorest neighbourhoods will, on average, die seven years earlier than people living in the richest neighbourhoods.'[65] If this model is to have positive results, governments and other agencies must be prepared to direct appropriate resources to empowering people to change.[66] Yet, governments so often want quick-fix solutions to the cultural causes of poor health and are not prepared to assign resources for the long haul.

In terms of the binary poles in the founding myth of healthcare this model mirrors the values of equity, social justice and community solidarity that are integral to the founding mission of healthcare.

Economic rationalist model

The remarkable increase of for-profit hospitals in the United States, particularly in the last three decades, provides an excellent example of an unregulated economic rationalist model of healthcare. Devotees of this model vigorously advocate the philosophy of 'small-government' and market-managed policies, for example, deregulation, privatization of government services, lower taxation and the significant reduction in government spending on welfare and other services for the poor. The primary aim of healthcare management, according to economic rationalists, is the financial return to shareholders, not the quality of service to patients. Nor are they concerned for the millions on the margins of society in poverty and/or without medical insurance. 'The business', not the 'the

65 The Marmot Review (2010) *Fair Society, Healthy Lives. Strategic Review of Health Inequalities in England post-2010 – Executive Summary*, p.10. Accessed 14 June 2012 at www.instituteofhealthequity.org. Michael Marmot, University College London, is a specialist in the social determinants of health.

66 See Linda J. Jones (1994) *The Social Context of Health and Health Work*. London: Macmillan, pp.32–38.

mission' now becomes the driving force in healthcare[67] (Figure 2.2) and the financial cost of fostering unbridled consumerism in healthcare to the nation is massive. It is conservatively estimated that unnecessary medical services in the United States account for one-third of medical costs, or some $700 billion. That is, the country 'could insure the uninsured seven times over with the amount of documented money wasted annually'.[68]

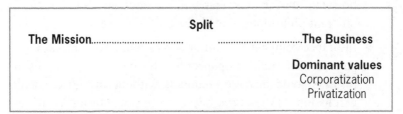

Figure 2.2: Economic rationalist model of healthcare

There has been the dramatic increase in what is called 'managed care' as a reaction to the rising costs of private healthcare in the United States in the form of insurance agencies that aim to reduce costs by controlling the choice of medical clinicians and hospitals.[69] One form of managed care is the health maintenance organization (HMO) which is a business, a medical provider and a form of health insurance all in one. The phenomenal increase in the number of HMOs and other forms of managed care is causing increasing anger for the following reasons: personal greed, not the values of solidarity and equity characteristic of the founding story of healthcare, is driving the market; the system fails to ensure that those most in need receive adequate healthcare; and there is no certitude that the introduction of market economics has led to a reduction in costs nor an improvement in health outcomes. Before President Obama's battle in 2009–2010 to extend healthcare, America was spending 18 per cent of its GDP on health, while more than 45 million people continued to lack any health insurance.[70] Great Britain, with its NHS that covers the entire nation, spends about half that amount.

67   See Relman 2010b, pp.15–67.
68   Guy Clifton (2009) 'Healing health care.' *America* (8–15 June), 12.
69   See Arbuckle 2000, pp.66–70.
70   Donald Dworkin estimates that 'the uninsured of working age have a 40 per cent higher risk of death than those who are privately insured'; (2012) 'Why the mandate is constitutional: The real argument.' *New York Review of Books 59*, 8, 4.

○ Prior to the rapid development of managed care companies beginning in the 1980s, hospitals in the United States ran their affairs on 'explicit and implicit understandings that allowed doctors and hospitals to balance professionalism, profitability, and service'.[71] Voluntary or non-profit hospitals historically received uninsured patients and did not insist that every action should be calculated according to its profitability. But for-profit hospitals, that are answerable to shareholders, hold a radically different philosophy, that is, the profit motive.

○ Insurance companies could now refuse to cover chronically ill patients and could drop people who became chronically ill. Insurers could increase premiums without any governmental permission. HMOs have been accused of refusing costly but necessary treatment and/or of sending patients home from hospitals before they are ready in order to cut costs and maintain profits. In 2000 one huge healthcare company, Aetna, Inc., cut 2 million of its 19 million customers and closed Medicare HMOs that were considered unprofitable.[72]

○ One advantage of HMOs and other types of managed care is that they compelled clinicians to agree to prearranged payment for their services and thus to be more publicly accountable.[73] However, contrary to their talk of 'cost-effectiveness' or 'reform', the primary feature of for-profit healthcare services is the consolidation of a major industry with the same aim as other industries, namely to return a profit. The American economic rationalist model of healthcare is diametrically opposed to the foundational model: healthcare is considered a commodity to be sold, not a basic social right. With the continuing development of expensive technological innovations healthcare is increasingly confined to those who can pay for it.

71 Robert Kuttner (1996) 'Columbia/HCA and the resurgence of the for-profit hospital business.' *New England Journal of Medicine 335*, 5, 362.
72 See M. Freudenheim (2000) 'Aetna to shed customers and jobs in effort to cut health care costs.' *The New York Times* (19 December), A1.
73 See Emily Friedman (1996) 'Capitation, integration, and managed care.' *Journal of the American Medical Association 275*, 12, 957–962.

USA: REFORM EFFORTS

In 1993 President Clinton attempted a radical reform of the healthcare system that demanded dramatic structural and attitudinal changes in the nation: healthcare should no longer be a luxury for the privileged and a 'fringe benefit' from employers, but only a wish for the ill-fated remainder of the population. He listed six goals in his healthcare reform plan: security, simplicity, savings, choice, quality and responsibility.[74] To provide all Americans with life-long healthcare security, his proposals included: a system of universal coverage according to the existing policy that employers must provide health insurance for employees; government aid to assist smaller businesses to build up this insurance system; restrictions to control the rising costs of healthcare, and a wider choice of physicians for consumers (something that many insurance companies had previously refused to accept).

His plan was rejected. Powerful lobby groups, such as the insurance companies, claimed that further government intervention was unnecessary because costs could be controlled and good quality achieved through increased, not less, competition.[75] Republican politicians refused to accept the fact that the deregulated market provision of healthcare had resulted in atrociously unjust costs to millions of people and to the nation as a whole. Lingering mythological fears about 'creeping socialism' in government once again emerged that made any rational debate on his plan impossible. Late in 1997, Clinton suggested a significantly altered plan, which included a 'patient's bill of rights', permitting people to receive emergency treatment and to choose a specialist without referral and expansion of Medicare to cover any 'near-elderly' who need early retirement. Republicans condemned the plan, claiming that it would lead to more government control (that is, in their terminology 'creeping socialism') and excessive costs.[76]

---

74   See 'American health care.' (1998) *The Economist* (7 March), 21–24.
75   See Wendy K. Mariner (1997) 'Business Versus Medical Ethics: Conflicting Standards for Managed Care.' In John W. Glasser and Ronald P. Hamel (eds) *Three Realms of Managed Care.* Kansas City, MO: Sheed and Ward, p.93.

In March 2010, despite massive opposition, President Obama signed into law a sweeping set of healthcare reforms under the title of the Patient Protection and Affordable Health Care Act. The Act had two main aims: first, to improve access to necessary healthcare for millions of uninsured and underinsured Americans, and second, to more successfully control healthcare costs so that access to necessary healthcare is more affordable for all citizens. The Act mandated coverage for 96 per cent of US citizens, including 36 million of those currently uninsured; approved federal subsidies to help people with low incomes afford the premiums; mandated employers to provide health insurance for workers with an exemption for small businesses; and set limitations on insurers, who could only sell policies that met government requirements, could no longer refuse coverage to people with pre-existing conditions, or drop policyholders who became seriously ill. The fundamental weakness of the reforms is that they still revolve around the profit-making insurance companies, which will be forever committed to keeping down costs and acquiring considerable wealth for themselves. And this will be done by denying or limiting treatment to patients. The opposition to the law has been, and continues to be, intense. By August 2011, 26 states had challenged the law[77] and a federal appeals court in Atlanta had concluded that it is unconstitutional to require everyone to buy insurance.[78] But on 26 July 2012 the Supreme Court narrowly upheld the centrepiece of Obama's healthcare reform that requires most citizens to obtain health insurance by 2014 or pay a financial penalty. However, the Court did substantially restrict one significant piece of the law that would have further expanded Medicaid, that is, the joint federal state programme providing healthcare to poor and disabled people.

---

76 See 'Health insurance.' (1997) *The Economist* (13 December), 31; Walter A. Zelman (1996) *The Changing Health Care Market Place*. San Francisco, CA: Jossey-Bass, pp.170–171, 216–217.

77 See David Cole (2011) 'Health care reform unconstitutional?' *The New York Review* (24 February), 9–11.

78 See 'Health reforms under attack.' (2011) *The Economist* (20 August), 32.

Welfare states: Myth shift and substitution

It is ironic that, while people in the United States struggle to extend healthcare services to the uninsured, that is, some form of universal healthcare, other countries are moving or have significantly already moved away from universal healthcare to the corporatization and privatization that have long characterized the American scene.

When the national health services of countries like Britain, New Zealand, Australia and Canada were established, their founding mythology embraced the values inherent in the Good Samaritan story. Healthcare was considered a fundamental human right, not something that should 'be bought or sold',[79] or subject to the vagaries of the marketplace. It was considered that healthcare should be provided by the state, paid for through taxation and access be guaranteed on the basis of need, not the ability to pay.

By the late 1970s and 1980s, however, these governments were increasingly confronted with serious questions about the financial sustainability of their healthcare systems, rising demands for choice, especially from wealthier middle classes and aging populations. Governments sought some quick solutions. They felt hampered by the proliferation of local boards jealously in control of their own hospitals. The solution? Apply the principles of the market economy and management to healthcare, with its primary focus on profit. Remove local accountability, introduce a competitive quasi-market system. Lay managers with industrial and commercial expertise were to control the medical professionals, and market forces were to influence significantly the allocation of services.[80] The false assumption underlying these 'solutions' is that healthcare can be easily transformed into a free, competitive market like any commercial business. Patients become consumers. It was also wrongly assumed that the managerial principle if 'you can't measure it, you can't manage it' could also be applied to healthcare. While some degree of measurement is possible and necessary, many areas of healthcare are impossible to determine statistically, especially the emotional and time aspects of caring for people.[81] The many failures of the US health system are enough to disprove these assumptions.

---

79   Pollock 2005, p.15.
80   Ibid., pp.36–131.
81   Pat and Hugh Armstrong (1998) *Universal Healthcare*. New York: New Press, p.140.

During the Thatcherite years in Britain, there was a deliberate effort at myth substitution in the NHS: the values of economic rationalism would gravely undermine the founding myth. Sir Keith Joseph, widely regarded as the founder of Thatcherism, 'called social justice a "will o' the wisp"', while, in 'the nineties, Dr Robin Harris (former Deputy Director of the Downing Street Policy Unit) castigated monasteries for their egalitarian habit of sharing'.[82] Not surprisingly, therefore, equity, for example, that is, equitable access based on need, not income, became increasingly undermined. Many poor people found that they now had to pay for optical care, prescriptions, dentistry and non-clinical hospital services. In brief, the New Right government in the United Kingdom, despite its rhetoric to the contrary, broke with the post-war democratic consensus that implicitly affirmed the foundational model of healthcare with its roots in the Good Samaritan mythological story.

In New Zealand the ideologically led neoliberal reforms were adopted with astounding speed. Hospitals were regarded as effective only if they resembled businesses and were conducted, as far as possible, for profit. Local boards were closed. Individuals were to have the primary responsibility for their healthcare; the state's role should steadily decrease. Welfare services were also drastically reduced. The consequences were disastrous – levels of poverty and social exclusion rose dramatically, with tragic results for the health of people on the margins.[83] In brief, the critical 'values such as human dignity, distributive justice, and social cohesion [were] given second place to the pursuit of efficiency, self-reliance, a fiscal balance, and a more limited state'.[84]

Two terms encapsulate this mythological change: corporatization and privatization. Corporatization means that healthcare institutions must be managed according to business principles. What does not pay should be closed. Competition between service providers will bring about the best results for patients. The 'twin concepts of choice and

---

82   See Davis *et al.* 2008, p.39.
83   See Christine Cheyne, Mike O'Brien and Michael Belgrave (2008) *Social Policy in Aotearoa New Zealand*, 4th edn. Melbourne: Oxford University Press, pp.232–233. In Australia likewise, health policy-makers gradually shifted their concern from equity and social justice to cost containment and cost-effectiveness.
84   Jonathan Boston and Paul Dalziel (1992) *The Decent Society?* Oxford: Oxford University Press, p.88.

competition',[85] that are so appealing to middle-class consumerism, are to be the guiding principles of decision-making. A healthcare facility has been described as resembling a garage for the repair of motor vehicles. People can choose what they consider to be the best medical repair shop.[86] Privatization means that hospitals and other healthcare services are transferred entirely, or in part, from public ownership to either not-for-profit or for-profit institutions. The more privatization occurs the less public accountability there is. For example, when services are outsourced to for-profit organizations they are accountable primarily to their shareholders, not the public.

Reacting in the late 1990s to the failures of neoliberalism in New Zealand, Australia and Britain, governments were forced to modify their laissez-faire policies by returning to some of the fundamental values of social democracy. Power returned to local authorities through the establishment of, for example, Foundation Trusts in England with a limited degree of democratic accountability,[87] the new District Health Boards in New Zealand[88] and to a more limited extent in Australia. In New Zealand the government slowly moved to prioritize quality over choice.[89] But the principles of market economics still remained to varying degrees. In England, for example, the government decided to use private financing in the NHS for the building of new hospitals (Private Finance Initiative), with disputed financial effectiveness.[90] In 2005 frontline staff, including clinicians, were being urged to be more creative in responding to patients' needs, 'freeing up the entrepreneurialism…and developing new types of provider organizations'.[91] In Britain, New Labour called this 'managing the market.' Victor Fuchs, a health economist, has argued that even in the United States, 'an intricate web of social, political,

85 Klein 2006, *The New Politics of the NHS*, 5th edn. Oxford: Radcliffe, p.257.
86 Ibid., p.254, and Alec Morton and Jocelyn Cornwell (2009) 'What's the difference between a hospital and a bottling factory?' *British Medical Journal 339*, 428–430.
87 See Alan Deacon (2008) 'Employment.' In Peter Alcock, Margaret May and Karen Rowlingson (eds) *The Student's Companion to Social Policy*. Oxford: Blackwell, p.322; Pollock 2005, pp.129–131; Rudolf Klein (2004) 'The first wave of NHS Foundation Trusts.' *British Medical Journal 328*, 1332.
88 See Robin Gauld (2009) *Revolving Doors: New Zealand's Health Reforms – The Continuing Saga*. Wellington, NZ: Health Services Research, pp.209–233.
89 See Cheyne *et al.* 2008, p.237.
90 See Pollock 2005, pp.27–30.
91 Department of Health 2005, p.15.

nomic considerations seems to preclude a pure *laissez-faire* approach to health.'[92]

In July 2010, however, the government in Westminster announced its intention to create the greatest reform of the NHS within England in a generation.[93] The reform, known as the Health and Social Care Act, was legislated by parliament in March 2012. The purpose is 'to create the largest and most vibrant social-enterprise sector in the world'.[94] The declared aim is to give patients more choice, to empower medical professions, to intensify competition and to increase efficiency in order to meet the needs of an ageing population, in ways that would control rising costs to the government. The NHS is to be liberated from management and handed to clinicians, resulting, it is claimed, in an estimated reduction in management costs of 45 per cent. That is, commissioning power is to be withdrawn from managers in primary care trusts (PCTs) and given instead to family doctors, who are to unite in consortia to purchase care for their patients. Doctors will no longer be accountable to ministers or the Department of Health, but to the patients and public they serve. At first sight the extensive reform is laudable, but a closer examination shows its ultimate aim is an intensification of the privatization of healthcare services. Few clinicians have either the time or expertise to manage 80 per cent of the NHS budget in order to buy hospitals or community services. This will open the way for huge for-profit organizations, mainly from the United Health, to organize the consortia. They will be accountable directly to their shareholders, not the patients or general public.[95]

---

92 Victor Fuchs (1994) *The Future of Health Policy*. Cambridge, MA: Harvard University Press, p.37.

93 Because of the political devolution of powers since the late 1990s, the Scottish Parliament and the National Assembly of Wales have substantially resisted the quasi-market reforms that characterize the NHS in England. See Harrison and McDonald 2008, pp.156–161.

94 See Department of Health 2010, p.8.

95 Nick Clegg, the Deputy Prime Minister and leader of the Liberal Democrats in the coalition government, vowed not to let the 'profit motive drive a coach and horses through the NHS' after party members voted to reject the reforms. Reported by Brian Wheeler (2011) 'Nick Clegg Vows to Protect NHS from "Profit Motive."' BBC News (12 March). Accessed 15 June 2012 at www.bbc.co.uk/news/uk-politics-12722836. See 'Where lucre is still filthy' 2011, 59–60.

Critique

There are several major criticisms of the economic rationalist model of healthcare. First, the gravest and most fundamental problem is that it is diametrically opposed to the founding mythology of healthcare. Julian Hart succinctly commented that the NHS was possible because there was in the first place 'a shared popular understanding of solidarity. If that understanding becomes replaced by consumerism, the NHS will have lost its foundations.'[96] The second criticism of market economics as an ideology is that it has failed.[97] The recent world economic crisis testifies to this. So, why should this ideology be trusted to work in healthcare? Some argue that choice and competition has improved care, efficiency and management.[98] Others disagree.[99] There is still scant evidence that private sector firms motivated by competition would necessarily produce more efficient and effective public sector institutions. One healthcare academic, commenting on the NHS, concluded: 'Most real improvements have been achieved by managerial action rather than competition.'[100] Competition in the United States, where economic rationalism has been at its extreme in healthcare, definitely leads to enormous wastage of resources in two main areas, namely in administration and in excess capacity of facilities, equipment and specialized personnel.[101]

Third, the emphasis on competition and choice as the driving forces in healthcare reform continues to reinforce the view that

96 Julian T. Hart (2006) *The Political Economy of Health Care: A Clinical Perspective.* Bristol: Policy Press, p.3.
97 See John R. Saul (1995) *The Unconscious Civilization.* New York: Penguin, p.122.
98 See Zack Cooper *et al.* (2011) 'Does hospital competition save lives? Evidence from the English NHS Patient Choice Reforms.' *Economic Journal 121*, 554 (August), 228–260.
99 See an overview of the debate by Penelope Dash and David Meredith (2010) 'When and how provider competition can improve health care delivery.' *McKinsey Quarterly.* Accessed at www.mckinseyquarterly.com. The authors comment that a study in 2002 discovered 'that competition among English hospitals may have worsened the quality of care in the UK National Health Service (NHS) to a small degree. A subsequent paper…reported that hospital competition did shorten waiting times, but it also appeared to have reduced care quality…' (p.2). John E. Wenneberg concludes that oversupply of services throughout the United States significantly adds to healthcare costs. See his book (2010) *Tracking Medicine: A Researcher's Quest to Understand Health Care.* New York: Oxford University Press, pp.119–169.
100 David Hands (2010) 'Inspiration, Ideology, Evidence and the National Health.' Lecture to the Welsh Institute for Health and Social Care (9 March), p.8. Accessed at www.sochealth.co.uk/news/hands.htm.
101 See Fuchs 1994, p.160. Back in 1966 there were 10,000 mammogram machines in the United States, when 2000 would fill existing demand; 5000 would in fact have screened the entire population.

healthcare is synonymous with hospitals, despite the fact that technology is leading to a reduction in the number of hospitals.[102] The health needs of the poor and vulnerable can be hidden from the concerns of the socioeconomically well-off sections of the population in the desire of the latter for choices in healthcare. So the Marmot Review concluded that the English NHS funding and effort has been distorted in favour of treatment in the acute sector.[103] And it is reported, that 'despite the presence of targets and central government rhetoric on reducing health inequalities, NHS staff at local levels viewed other priorities as much more important, for example...achieving financial balance in NHS trusts'.[104] In 2004 the government did target 70 local authorities and primary health trusts with the worst health and deprivation records to provide more resources, but more than half of England's deprived population was overlooked.[105] The fact is that health inequalities have widened since 1997.[106] With the removal of PCTs there is now even less certainty that health needs, including housing and employment, will feature significantly in the decisions of doctors' consortia.

Fourth, the use of the term 'customer' is obviously not entirely accurate because consumers of healthcare 'do not have the expertise to make informed choices about their treatment'.[107] There is a duty to give patients as much information as possible, but ultimately there is a limit to the amount of expertise they can absorb, unless they themselves become medical professionals! People, especially on the margins, do not have the resources to make choices or participate in decision-making.[108] Patients, according to Angela Coulter writing in the *British Medical Journal*, are more concerned about the quality of care, values such as respect and empathy, than about structural or

---

102 See Norman Vetter (1995) *The Hospital: From Centre of Excellence to Community Support.* London: Chapman and Hall, pp.1–4.

103 See Marmot Review 2010, p.85. Only four per cent of NHS funding in England in 2010 is being directed to prevention.

104 King's Fund (2010) *A High-Performing NHS? A Review of Progress 1997-2010.* London: King's Fund, p.81. Accessed 15 June 2012 at www.kingsfund.org.uk/publications/a_highperforming_nh.html.

105 Marmot Review 2010, p.87.

106 See King's Fund 2010, pp.77–87.

107 Steve Taylor and David Field (1997) *Sociology of Health and Health Care.* Oxford: Blackwell, p.37.

108 See Deacon 2008, p.324, and Chris Yuill, Iain Crinson and Edith Duncan (2010) *Key Concepts in Health Studies.* London: Sage Publications, pp.175–178.

financial reform.[109] Fifth, significant areas of healthcare can never be measured in financial terms, for example, the treatment for mental illnesses. Finally, privatization favours the situation in which private healthcare facilities can 'cherry pick' the most profitable cases and leave the less profitable to the public system.

However, to repeat the major criticism of the economic rationalist model is its distortion of the founding mythology of healthcare. The primary emphasis becomes less and less on the values of 'the mission'. The values of 'the business' dominate. The holistic needs of patients, especially the poor, are increasingly put to one side. The poor have no muscle to battle the hegemonic political and economic power of the socially and economically well-off, and the present reforms with their emphasis on choice and competition further reinforces their powerlessness. There is no sustained effort to reach out to the less fortunate in England.

Summary

○ This chapter has highlighted conflict between the values inherent in healthcare: the tension between 'the mission' on the one hand, with values of human dignity, compassion, solidarity, equity and social justice, and 'the business' of healthcare on the other, with values of individualism, efficiency, cost-effectiveness, key performance indicators and demanding targets.[110] The mission pole of the tension must be the driving force in all healthcare policies and implementation.

○ The social model of healthcare emphasizes values of the mission pole of the founding myth, but the biomedical and economic rationalist models are in conflict with the founding story of healthcare. The more governments continue to encourage the rhetoric of individual choice and competition, the more people will be unwilling to support taxation increases for a national

---

109 See Angela Coulter (2005) 'The NHS revolution: Health care in the market place – what do patients and the public want from primary care?' *British Medical Journal 331* (19 November), 1199–1201.

110 See Rudolf Klein (2002) 'A Babel of Voices: Values, Policy-Making and the NHS.' In Bill New and Julia Neuberger (eds) *Hidden Assets: Values and Decision-Making in the NHS.* London: King's Fund, pp.33–59.

system that responds proactively to the needs of people on the margins of society. Bryan Turner's assessment of the Australian healthcare scene in 1995 could well be applied now to England: '[The] social struggle over...disease is a political conflict over the distribution of power...The dynamics of welfare distribution, for example of health-care arrangements, are the outcome of conflicts between elite groups for the control...of resources.'[111] In the healthcare debate, individualism and individual self-interest are increasingly winning in England, to the detriment of the common good. In the United States, the recent reform in favour of a more equitable healthcare system is under severe attack from pro-economic rationalist politicians.

○ No government can allow the costs of healthcare to continue to spiral. The two most significant reasons for the escalating expenses of healthcare are emerging medical technologies and the rapid growth of elderly populations. Hence, we face more rigorous rationing of resources and/or higher taxes. Both are politically unpopular. However rationing is done, the real challenge is to decide the criteria on which decisions are made. There are no simple ways of establishing these criteria.[112] The fundamental issue remains a philosophical or moral question. What kind of a society does a nation seek – one that maximizes the quality of life for the most productive, *or* one that draws the weakest closer to the standards of the strongest? If the first is chosen, then medical services will tend, as is especially noticeable in the United States, towards increasingly expensive technology and medicine, while the second will focus on community or the common good.

○ Unless this question is openly debated and addressed, then rationing will be directed according to pragmatic exigencies based on a philosophy that may be destructive of the common good. It is time to reconnect healthcare with its founding values. Healthcare cannot be reformed, or costs controlled, without changing some deeply held underlying values. We need a cultural revolution committed to re-finding and

---

111 Turner 1995, p.84.
112 See Butler 1999, pp.5–39.

implementing the foundational values of the NHS.[113] In the words of Robert Francis, when presenting his official inquiry into the Mid Staffordshire NHS Foundation Trust[114] in 2010:

> People must always come before numbers. Individual patients and their treatment are what really matters. Statistics, benchmarks and action plans are tools, not ends in themselves. They should not come before patients and their experiences. This is what must be remembered by all those who design and implement policy for the NHS.[115]

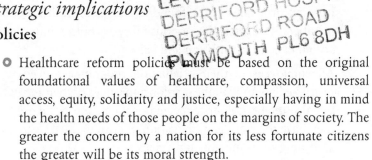

Strategic implications

Policies

○ Healthcare reform policies must be based on the original foundational values of healthcare, compassion, universal access, equity, solidarity and justice, especially having in mind the health needs of those people on the margins of society. The greater the concern by a nation for its less fortunate citizens the greater will be its moral strength.

○ Reforms of this kind require committed and skilled leaders at all levels of health systems who are able to rearticulate the founding values and implement them through appropriate policies and actions.

Implementation

○ Political leaders have the obligation to state clearly the foundational values that should be underpinning their policy decisions. At times there is bound to be conflict between values, for example, between the demands of equity and universal access. In this situation governments are obliged to explain why there is a conflict and invite citizens to help resolve the issue

---

113 See Callahan 2009, pp.5, 7.
114 See Francis 2010.
115 Robert Francis, Accessed on 11 November 2010 at www.midstaffsinquiry.com/pressrelease. html.

through open debate. This is an exercise of true leadership, characterized by a refusal to be swayed by influential people's wants rather than the authentic health needs of the general population.

○ Citizens collectively and individually have the right and duty to challenge governments to be true to the founding values of healthcare.

○ Administrators of healthcare institutions, for example, CEOs, will involve their executive staffs in defining the mission of their institutions based on the founding values of healthcare; all decisions will then need to be informed according to adult learning principles of the founding values of healthcare. Staff members have then the responsibility to hold administrators accountable to the mission and values.

○ All employees in their orientation programmes need to be instructed not only in the mission and values of their institution but also the behaviours expected of them, and be advised that they have the right and obligation to critique their institutions according to its mission and values.

CHAPTER 3

Tribalism between Clinicians and Managers

Risk to Patients

> *Culture controls the manager more than the manager controls culture.*
>
> *(Edgar H. Schein)*[1]

This chapter explains:

- that tribal-like tensions can exist between medical and management subcultures

- that historical factors and the qualities of the two subcultures have inevitably fostered mutual antagonism

- that among the symptoms of the tensions are unarticulated grief on the part of clinicians, feuding and 'subcultural splitting'

- that for the safety and welfare of patients teamwork must develop across the tribal boundaries.

To speak of tribal tensions in healthcare institutions may sound rather exaggerated. However, the author of the commission inquiring into the crises within the acute care services of the public health system of New South Wales, Australia, concluded that 'one impediment to good, safe care which infects the whole public hospital system is the breakdown of good working relations between [medical] clinicians and management which is very detrimental to patients'. Distrust and deep antipathies divide the two groups. In an effective but frightening analogy, he likened the breakdown to the Great Schism, the lasting split between the Eastern and Western Christian Churches in 1045, when each side accused the other of having fallen victim to heresy

---

1   Schein 1985, p.314.

and having started the division. The commission concluded that the schism in the health system is 'alienating the most skilled in the medical workforce from service in the public system'.[2]

The purpose of this chapter is to examine this dramatic division between clinicians, particularly medical clinicians, and managers in healthcare institutions. Although much has been written on this problem by sociologists and management experts, this chapter aims to clarify the reasons for the persistent split between medical clinicians and managers from a cultural anthropological perspective. The problem is not unique to Australia. It is a worldwide phenomenon and both parties have been described as deeply unhappy with the tension.[3] There has even been talk of mass resignations by general practitioners from the NHS in England, one major reason being their dissatisfaction with managers, who, they feel, are invading their professional territory. Serious discontent commonly exists also among managers who complain that medical clinicians are financially naive and unwilling to acknowledge the immense complexity of contemporary healthcare institutions. Many feel unfairly scapegoated by clinicians and politicians for the inadequacies of the public health systems.[4]

The schism-like behaviour is both a cause and an effect of the mutual discontent. Although, within the complex culture of a healthcare institution, there are many other subcultures such as nurses, physiotherapists, radiographers, and medical laboratory scientific officers and hospital social workers,[5] the dominant subcultures in tension are those of clinicians and managers. They impact on every other healthcare subculture.

2   Garling 2008b, p.11.
3   See Richard Smith (2001) 'Why are doctors so unhappy?' *British Medical Journal 322* (5 May), 1073–1074, and Nigel Edwards, Mary J. Kornack and Jack Silversin (2002) 'Unhappy doctors: What are the causes and what can be done?' *British Medical Journal 324* (6 April), 835–838.
4   See Greener 2009, pp.239–244; Huw T.O. Davies and Stephen Harrison (2003) 'Trends in doctor–manager relationships.' *British Medical Journal 326* (22 March); Paul Fitzsimmons and Tony White (1997) 'Medicine and management: A conflict facing general practice.' *Journal of Management in Medicine 11*, 3, 124–131; Peter Degeling *et al.* (2003) 'Medicine, management, and modernization: A "danse macabre"?' *British Medical Journal 326* (22 March), 649–652; Peter Degeling and Adrian Carr (2004) 'Leadership for the systemization of health care: The unaddressed issue in health care reform.' *Journal of Health Organization and Management 18*, 6, 399–414.
5   See James Drife and Ian Johnston (1995) 'Handling the conflicting cultures in the NHS.' *British Medical Journal 310* (22 April), 1054–1056.

Evolution of tensions

In Chapter 2 it was explained that the medical profession's loss of its dominant position in hospital administration has led to significant strained relationships between medical clinicians and managers. However, to better appreciate the reasons for the rise of the divisive tension it is helpful to review the historical development of the hospital system. The rationale of the growth of the medical profession's hegemonic dominance until recent times then becomes apparent. Five stages of development can be identified. First, there was the *monastic* period, up to the time of the dissolution of the monasteries under Henry VIII in England. Religious institutions provided care for the sick, especially the poor, and safe havens for travellers.[6] The *refuge* stage of hospital development took place between the mid-seventeenth century and the late 1920s. During this period hospitals were little more than refuges for the sick and destitute, the well-off being cared for in their homes. Medical knowledge was poor and much of the treatment offered was in fact harmful to patients. However, boards of trustees, not medical clinicians, administered these mostly non-profit institutions and raised money from the community to support them. By the late 1920s there were approximately 7000 hospitals in the United States.[7]

In the *physician* stage (from early 1930s to the mid-1960s) power moved from trustees and community control to medical staff. With the discovery of powerful new drugs hospitals were able to focus primarily on treating patients rather than just caring for them. Physicians controlled the knowledge and technologies, giving them very significant organizational and political power over larger and more complex hospitals. As the practice of medicine became more scientific the biomedical model of healthcare flourished. The training of medical clinicians reflected this scientific and technological focus, with little or no emphasis being given to person-to-person communication and management skills. A *Lancet* survey conducted in 1996 found that only 45 per cent of medical clinicians in the study considered they had acquired satisfactory training in communication

6   See Vetter 1995, pp.4–5.
7   See Dennis D. Pointer and Charles M. Ewell (1994) *Really Governing: How Health System and Hospital Boards Can Make a Difference.* Albany, NY: Delmar, pp.4–5.

skills, although all felt they had received adequate education in the diagnosis and management of diseases. Almost half felt they lacked the skills to relate to the human and personal aspects of their work; that is, they considered themselves to be poorly equipped to relate to the narratives of patients,[8] and by implication to personnel around them.

The *business* stage developed from the mid-1960s through the mid-1980s as hospitals became more specialized. Since the business stage demanded far more commercial acumen, lay administrators were introduced, but only as assistants to medical clinicians who continued to maintain control over hospitals. The *corporate* stage began in the mid-1980s and continues to this day, in response to the need for hospitals to survive financially in the face of increasing competition and their ever-increasing complexity. This is the period in which economic rationalism starts to flourish not just in the United States, but also in Britain and elsewhere. This is the stage of the dual processes of managerialism and internal markets, with their emphasis on such issues as output targets and monetary incentives, accompanied by the declining influence of doctors. This is 'government by the market', that is, health policy is removed from the political arena and placed into the market 'rendering any claims on public heath care subject to the discourse of management, efficiency, and competition'.[9] In countries like Britain, New Zealand, Canada and Australia, managers increasingly have been required to develop a more corporate outlook, as governments demanded that their institutions reach set performance financial targets. Managers were now seen 'more as agents of governments than as facilitators of professionally driven agendas'.[10] In the United States, managed care processes expanded immensely under the direction of health insurance companies, with their aim of reducing costs by control of patients' choice of doctors and hospitals. Doctors who join managed care plans are paid at lower rates, but benefit from having a definite number of patients. Of course, in the process the autonomy of doctors has diminished, becoming increasingly under the control

---

8   See A.J. Ramirez *et al.* (1996) 'Mental health of hospital consultants: The effects of stress and satisfaction at work.' *The Lancet 347* (16 March), 724–728.

9   John Germov (1998) 'Challenges to Medical Dominance.' In John Germov (ed.) *Second Opinion: An Introduction to Health Sociology.* Melbourne: Oxford University Press, p.244.

10 Davies and Harrison 2003, p.646.

of lay people.[11] Accordingly, the operational and strategic decision-making in hospitals slipped away from clinicians in a relatively brief period of time. Managers were to become, in their own right, a new, separate, non-clinical profession. The stage was set for conflict.

Models

While this brief historical overview helps to explain a fundamental cause of the tensions between medical clinicians and managers, there are other contributing factors. For example, the difference between medical professionals and managers is not just confined to the fact that the former generally commit themselves to a life-long profession, and the latter do not necessarily do so. More profoundly, they think and feel differently about their work because they belong to two quite separate subcultures in the wider culture of healthcare. The two subcultures are so mythologically diverse (see Figure 3.1) that the 'potential for conflict arising from cultural differences is almost limitless'.[12] The inter-tribal tension is now viewed through the lens of four models, namely the 'culture clash', 'unarticulated cultural grief', 'subcultural feuding' and 'cultural splitting' models. However, readers need to be mindful that a culture model is an anthropological construct that does not claim perfectly to mirror reality. Nuanced explanations or details are omitted in order allow us to grasp a little more clearly what is in fact a highly complex situation. Any particular culture is then compared with the model to see the extent of the resemblances.

Model 1: Culture clash

As explained in Chapter 1, a culture or subculture is a pattern of meanings encased in a network of symbols, myths, narratives and rituals. Individuals and subdivisions create these patterns, as they

---

11   In reaction to the managed care control of doctors some physicians organized to own hospitals themselves in the United States. However, the Obama healthcare reform forbade physician-owned hospitals from expanding or undertaking new construction. This affected about 300 hospitals. This affected 300 hospitals. The American Medical Association (AMA), the physicians well-financed union, vigorously opposed the Obama reform, because the organization feared that doctors would lose further independence and would have to be more accountable to the public. The economist, Jeff Madrick, commented: 'The AMA called White House staffers followers of the Moscow party line.' See Jeff Madrick (2012) 'Obama and healthcare: The straight story.' *The New York Review 59*, 11 (21 June), 46.

12   Drife and Johnston 1995, p.1054.

struggle to respond to the competitive pressures of power and limited resources in a rapidly globalizing and fragmenting world. This pattern instructs its adherents about what is considered to be the correct way to feel, think and behave. In view of this definition, two points are relevant.

First, tension and conflict are inevitable between the two subcultures because they must compete for power and control over limited resources available to healthcare institutions. Second, people of one subculture are apt to view other subcultures as inferior to their own, expressing their ethnocentric superior distaste in prejudicial stereotypes. A stereotype is a preformed image or picture that we have of things or people; it is a shorthand, but faulty, method of handling or grasping a complex world. By placing things and people into preformed categories, I feel I am controlling a world that threatens my desired sense of order or meaning. Prejudices do not consist only of stereotypes; rather they are stereotypes motivated by strong, and often powerful, impulses of feeling that force the prejudiced person to see only what he or she wants to see, even to see things that are not there at all. Hence, occupational prejudice can be defined as 'an antipathy based upon a faulty and inflexible generalization. It may be felt or expressed. It may be directed toward a group as a whole, or toward an individual because he [sic] is a member of that group.'[13] These dynamics are evident in the subcultural divisions between clinicians and management; divisive stereotypes of one another abound.[14] One simple indication of this is noted by two observers of the NHS who concluded several years ago that it 'is rare for doctors and managers to enjoy lunch or a tea break together, except at formal meetings'.[15] This lack of informal common rituals illustrates the depth of the culture divide. At times, managers' efforts to collaborate with medical clinicians can be hampered when clinicians are part-time consultants to hospitals but are not employed by them. Managers are reluctant to insist on the contractual obligations of the clinicians for fear that the latter will leave for sole private practice.[16]

---

13   Gordon Allport (1958) *The Nature of Prejudice*. New York: Doubleday, p.10.
14   See comments by Huw Davies, Claire-Louise Hodges and Thomas G. Rundall (2003) 'Views of doctors and managers on doctor–manager relationship in the NHS.' *British Medical Journal* 326 (22 March), pp.626–628.
15   Ibid.
16   See NSW Independent Panel (2009) *Independent Panel: Caring Together: The Health Action Plan for NSW State 1 Progress Report (October 2009)*. Sydney: NSW Independent Panel, p.30.

	Clinicians	Managers
Focus	Individual patients	Systems/groups/populations
Identity	Profession	Organization
Patients	Close	Remote
Commitment	Life-long profession	Often short-term
Style	Individualistic	Collaborative
Authority source	Expertise	Positional/bureaucratic
Power application	Inclination to dictate	Preference: negotiation/ delegation
Judgment base	Scientific-research	Weak objective verification
Structure	Network-oriented	Hierarchical/bureaucratic
Planning	Short-term	Long-term
Accountability	Patients/professional bodies	Government/general public
Chaos	'Avoid'	'Embrace'

Figure 3.1: Subcultural clashing qualities

The immediate operative myths and values in these subcultures differ quite radically (see Figure 3.1).[17] As explored in Chapter 1, myths are deeply embedded, emotionally charged narratives that guide our feeling, thinking and behaviour. The operative myth for clinicians is their focus on the needs of individual patients to whom they are primarily accountable for their actions.[18] To maintain this focus, they expect to have sufficient resources allocated to them, but there is the persistently strong feeling that managers are refusing to respond appropriately. Managers know that resources are limited, and for this reason their immediate operative myth is very different indeed. Doctors are anxious about patient outcomes, whereas managers must

---

17 See Marie L. Thorne (1997) 'Myth-management in the NHS.' *Journal of Management in Medicine 11,* 3, 172, and the particularly helpful overview by Paul Parkin (2009) *Managing Change in Healthcare: Using Action Research.* London: Sage Publications, pp.56–60.

18 Thomas H. Lee, reflecting on the American situation, concludes that cultural barriers to change in healthcare, such as the doctors' opposition to being accountable to management, their hesitancy to criticize fellow-doctors, their dislike of teamwork, 'reflect a deep-seated belief that physician autonomy is crucial to quality in health care.' Thomas H. Lee (2010) 'Turning doctors into leaders.' *Harvard Business Review 88,* 4, 58.

be concerned 'about patient experience (which includes outcomes, but only as part of a mix to be met out of finite resources)'.[19]

With the rapid development of medical technology, however, doctors are increasingly concerned not only with the medical needs of the whole human person as such, but also with particular aspects of the person. This increase in specialization has a further consequence. It is leading to the development of what might be called 'sub-subcultures' within the wider medical subculture. The medical profession is, in reality, a very divided one, with minimal corporate identity and little feeling of belonging, for example, to the NHS in Britain. Different specialities have their own colleges; in Britain, for example, we find colleges such as the Royal College of General Practitioners and the Royal College of Physicians. These sub-subcultures have been termed 'medical silos',[20] that is, groups of specialists who keep to themselves, are overly sensitive to the importance of hierarchical status, and discourage the sharing of information with other professional silos.[21] This jealously guarded individualism is inimical to the development of teamwork among themselves,[22] across the silo barriers, between themselves and nurses, and between themselves and managers. Because of this individualism, the degree of mutual support among medical clinicians is poor. Little wonder that many experience high levels of unaddressed stress and 'seem to deny the effect of stress and fatigue on performance',[23] further discouraging them from openly acknowledging and discussing their medical errors with their colleagues (see Guideline 3, Chapter 1). For this reason, the Garling Report into the acute care services of the public hospitals in New South Wales concluded that a 'new model of teamwork will be required to replace the old individual and independent "silos" of professional care'.[24]

The individualistic focus of clinicians is contrary to the operative myth that characterizes the work of managers. To be effective,

---

19   Nigel Edwards *et al.* (2003) 'Doctors and managers: A problem without a solution.' *British Medical Journal 326* (22 March), 609.

20   See Garling 2008b, p.4.

21   See Henry Mintzberg (2009) *Managing.* Harlow: Pearson, pp.169–170.

22   See J. Bryan Sexton, Eric J. Thomas and Robert L. Helmreich (2000) 'Error, stress, and teamwork in medicine and aviation: Cross sectional surveys.' *British Medical Journal 320* (18 March), 745–749.

23   Ibid., p.745.

24   See Garling 2008b, p.4.

managers must concentrate on many different groups withir
outside their institutions, viewing them not as isolated unit
as integrated into wider organizational systems. On the one hand,
doctors require scientific evidence in decision-making, but managers
are rarely able to achieve such certainty in their work when the
financial, administrative and policy decisions from governments are
in constant flux. Managers must ask and answer questions like: What
are the health needs of an entire health system? What should be the
priorities when resources are limited? Often managers must 'ponder
ambiguous issues collectively',[25] always sensitive to the fact that
their decisions might well have to change dramatically for reasons
beyond their control. Unions could suddenly go on strike, machinery
break down, new technology be installed or government health
departments may introduce new policies and financial restraints.

In summary, managers need constantly to struggle to maintain
a level of substantial order in the midst of constant uncertainty,
even chaos, if the healthcare systems are to respond to patients'
needs. This can be a frustrating task. Yet doctors are expected to
make crucial decisions in the here and now, allowing little room
for uncertainty. Management expert Henry Mintzberg commented
that, in the culture of medicine, practitioners are interventionists,
that is, their involvement with patients is normally intermittent and
crisis-oriented. Managers, however, must be about 'continuous and
pre-emptive care – to steady operations and sustain strategic positions
– more than intermittent, specialized, and radical cure'.[26] Their role
demands teamwork, having to be less hierarchical than doctors if
collaboration is to be achieved. Ultimately, the type of power for the
two groups is radically different: for managers, it is position power
within a bureaucratic system, but for doctors the most common
source of power is their professional expertise.[27]

Psychiatrist Anton Obholzer claimed that the Thatcherite style
of management in Britain's healthcare systems gave managers more
latitude not to have to consult with clinicians because it was thought
to be a waste of time and therefore inefficient. This top-down
approach viewed dialogue and cooperation between different sectors

---

25   Mintzberg 2009, p.120.
26   Ibid.
27   See relevant comments by Ellen Annandale (1998) *The Sociology of Health and Medicine: A Critical Introduction.* Oxford: Polity Press, pp.223–250.

of healthcare to be out of date. Obholzer examined the effects of not involving medical staff in the detail of budgets or financial management of the healthcare system. It encouraged doctors to share with the public and media the fantasy that if only they had unlimited health funds there would be nothing they could not do. This fostered a culture in which medical staff could consider themselves to be professionally omnipotent and that all failures were caused by heartless managers and insufficient resources.[28]

Culture shock reactions

The dynamics of culture shock are common throughout healthcare institutions and further help to explain the reactions of clinicians and managers when they are in contact with each other's subculture. The term 'culture shock', in general, is a label for a wide variety of different possible affective responses to culture-contact stress, which may include disorientation, depression, apathy, irrational or inappropriate responses. More particularly it is a reaction that can be blind and unreasoned, a reaction that is but a subconscious flight or escape from a culturally disagreeable environment. Three common symptoms of culture shock are the irrational refusal to understand the other culture, the urge to reassert the superiority of one's own cultural grouping and the deep-seated suspicion of the other culture.[29] These symptoms characterize the subcultures of managers and clinicians.

Model 2: Unarticulated cultural grief

Grief is experienced by groups and organizations as well as by individuals. It is the sorrow, anger, denial, guilt and confusion that so often accompany significant loss. Yet unless the cultures of groups and organizations acknowledge that loss in rituals of grieving and formally letting go, they – and the individuals within them – remain haunted by or trapped in the past, unable to open themselves to new ways of thinking and acting. Rightly did the Roman poet Ovid

---

28   See Anton Obholzer (1996) 'Managing Social Anxieties in Public Sector Organizations.' In Anton Obholzer and Vega Z. Roberts (eds) *The Unconscious at Work: Individual and Organizational Stress in the Human Services.* London: Routledge, pp.169–178.

29   See helpful analysis by Colleen Ward, Stephen Bochner and Adrian Furnham (2001) *The Psychology of Culture Shock.* Hove: Routledge.

claim that 'suppressed grief suffocates'.[30] Unarticulated grief remains like a powder-keg waiting to be ignited into all kinds of individual and community destructive behaviour.

Healthcare cultures are prone to experience overwhelming suppressed grief. They undergo change after change, with little or no chance for people and their institutions to ritualize their sense of loss. I was first alerted to this when I conducted a workshop for senior medical clinicians on personally coping with grief in their professional lives. To my surprise several present tearfully described how they had constantly to ignore their feelings of loss. No one had ever asked them how they felt when, no matter how hard they tried, they could not save the lives of their patients. Others spoke of the pain and anger they felt when essential staff had been assigned elsewhere in order to meet budget targets. One participant summed up the feelings of others when he said: 'Why does no one ever ask us how we feel when we experience loss? Why do we have to keep silent? It drains our energies.'

Psychoanalyst Wildred Bion uncovered a method to examine the inner processes of the cultures of healthcare facilities.[31] Healthcare institutions exist to protect people from loss and fear, so there is an added reason for these institutions and personnel not to openly acknowledge their own experience of loss. Obholzer,[32] explaining Bion's thinking, wrote that in the unconscious section of our being we have no comprehension of health, but we do have a concept of death. To keep in check our anxieties about death, we repress them, 'pushing down' these undesirable impulses deep down into the unconscious. We develop various defences that include the shaping of various institutions and rituals as part of this self-protective approach. All cultures manage these anxieties that death and loss evoke in different ways. In Christianity, for example, death is seen as a shift to a higher life in Christ (1 Cor. 15:54–55). With the growth of secularism, however, this understanding of death fails to provide meaning to many people. Now the fear of death is kept

---

30 Ovid, *Tristia*, book V, eleg.1, line 63. For an understanding of the significant relationship between ritual, grieving and organizational cultural change, see Gerald A. Arbuckle (1991) *Grieving for Change*. London: Geoffrey Chapman.

31 See Wilfred Bion (1967) *Second Thoughts*. London: Heinemann; Lyth 1988.

32 See Obholzer 1996, pp.170–171; Arbuckle 2000, pp.126–127.

under control by such institutions as hospitals and medical staff, the postmodern substitutes for the churches and their ritual leaders. Healthcare institutions and professions cannot provide the transition to a new life beyond death, but, in the collective unconscious, they are able to manage our fears about death and loss. For this reason 'our health service might more accurately be called a "keep-death-at-bay"'.[33] There is a common fantasy that hospitals and their staff (and even the national healthcare services themselves) will guard us from death. They will find the right medical ritual or solution to life-threatening illnesses and ageing. If they do not, they will have been unsuccessful in their mission. Patients and medical personnel can conspire together in creating this fantasy 'to protect the former from facing their fear of death and the latter from facing their fallibility'.[34]

This analysis of grief may help to explain some of the intensity of negative feelings on the part of clinicians towards managers. When universal healthcare was established in New Zealand, Australia and Britain, governments accepted the biomedical model of healthcare, the ascendancy of the medical profession, with its right to set its own standards, discipline offenders, control information to the public and the subordination of managers.[35] Dramatically, in the mid-1980s, this cosy relationship with governments changed. Within a short space of time, the medical profession lost considerable power and prestige. In Britain, for example, following the Griffiths Report in 1983,[36] with little or no consultation with the medical profession, 'chief executors' replaced senior doctors in the management of hospitals, with the task of assessing the performance of doctors and instilling in them the principle of value for money. The power base of doctors was now challenged from two sides: increased government regulation,[37] supported by a daunting array of new statistics, and the

---

33   Obholzer 1996, p.171.
34   Ibid.
35   See Oliver Morgan (1998) *Who Cares? The Great British Health Debate.* Oxford: Radcliffe Medical Press, p.17.
36   See David Cox (1992) 'Crisis and Opportunity in Health Service Management.' In Ray Loveridge and Ken Starkey (eds) *Continuity and Crisis in the NHS.* Buckingham: Open University Press..
37   Ian Greener (2009, p.233) comments on the situation in Britain: 'from the 1980s onwards the state has increasingly imposed policy rather than consulting with the doctors, and the medical profession has found itself excluded particularly from the policy formulation process'.

discipline of competition in a quasi-market.[38] Since then, more and more managerial and organizational reforms have further weakened the professional medical dominance and autonomy.[39] Managerialism became the government-led ideology, 'emphasizing targets, protocols, performance measurements and evidence-based decision making'.[40] Managerialism is an ideology that shapes ideas about what the NHS should be and how it should be structured and organized. Although autonomy significantly remained with the medical profession in particular areas within certain boundaries, such as the control over diagnosis and treatment,[41] the balance of power inexorably moved from doctors to managers (see the economic rationalist model, Chapter 2).[42] But clinicians, as ritual leaders of institutions that 'keep-death-at-bay', are not used to acknowledging failure in their professional lives. Hence, according to this hypothesis, they are ill prepared to face their loss of prestige and power. They suppress this unarticulated grief. Anger towards managers and governments is one of its symptoms. If clinicians, in particular, could ritually and regularly name their grief over loss of power and prestige, and let it go, it would help to release at least some of their suppressed personal and subcultural anger and sadness. This ritual cathartic action would provide opportunities for new expressions of creative cooperation between clinicians and managers to begin.

Model 3: Subcultural feuding

A basic assumption in this book is that the speed and pressures of constant change in healthcare creates persistent organizational cultural chaos, but 'one can neither work nor play nor theorize with chaos. Pure chaos is pure terror. One must find forms and frames within which to contain it.'[43] People and healthcare institutions must constantly cope with the pressures of cultural change and chaos. One way of coping is for ritual feuding to develop between rival groups. Anthropologically, a feud is defined as relations of mutual animosity

---

38   See Pollock 2005, pp.39–40.
39   Ibid., p.142.
40   Parkin 2009, p.76.
41   See Davies and Harrison 2003, p.647.
42   See Hunter 2002, p.73.
43   C. Fred Alford (1995) 'The group as a whole or acting out the missing leader.' *International Journal of Group Psychotherapy 45*, 1, 133.

between intimate groups in which a resort to limited violence – physical and/or verbal – is anticipated on both sides.[44] Feuding is thus a way of channelling physical or verbal violence through ritual so that an uneasy peace is maintained between hostile groups. Certain Eskimo societies cope with cultural chaos by breaking up into subcultural groups that resemble the *strong group/strong grid* model as devised by Mary Douglas (see Guideline 3, Chapter 1). These mutually antagonistic groups arrange what is called *nith*-song contests, which permit both sides to air their grievances in an open arena, but only by way of song and dance. After both sides have abused each other in melody and movement and finally collapsed into exhaustion, one side will emerge with more public acclaim than the other, but both have had the chance to give vent to their tensions, although always within safe limits.[45] The relationship that prevailed between the former Soviet Union and the United States, or between contemporary North and South Korea, could be classed as feuding. Of course, although the feuding parties present a united front, they will at the same time be internally divided by all kinds of rivalries and jealousies. These internal divisive behaviours are, however, temporarily suspended in order to cope with the external threats. The role of leaders in these sect-like groupings is to patrol the boundaries to ensure that authenticity is maintained and that outsiders who could contaminate their groups with dangerous thinking are kept out.

This model of feuding helps to explain how tensions are managed between the medical profession and management subcultures in healthcare institutions. Given the wider national and global chaos of healthcare, the two subcultures of medical clinicians and management each present united behaviour patterns of *strong group/strong grid* cultures to the general public, even though internally they may be divided. Every now and then, the representatives of both groups publicly and ritually feud with one another in the mass media, each claiming to have right on their side. Both groups in different ways feel threatened by the wider chaos of healthcare. Clinicians bond tightly with clinicians when threatened by a common foe, and managers with managers, both camps deeply distrustful of each

---

44   See Jacob Black-Michard (1975) *Feuding Societies*. Oxford: Basil Blackwell.
45   See Simon Roberts (1979) *Order and Dispute*. Harmondsworth: Pelican, pp.59–60.

other. Consequently, their separate groupings develop symptoms of sect-like behaviour. In Britain, the medical profession, having lost its dominant power in these systems through successive government decisions since the mid-1980s, has 'become increasingly vociferous and strident in their condemnation of the NHS in general and the cult of managerialism in particular'.[46] Some physicians view colleagues who take on management roles as 'traitors' or as having 'copped out'.[47] Many feel their traditional power is also being undermined in other ways. In common with Australia, New Zealand and other Western countries, some feel that the pressure to have nurses take over some of their responsibilities is further intruding on their professionalism.[48] Some would like more rigid demarcation rituals to keep non-physicians like nurses and midwives in their traditional roles. Then, there is the perceived threat of the increasing popularity of alternative medicines. Other clinicians are offended that they are being encouraged to adopt entrepreneurial and management skills. The more they do so, they claim, the more they lose contact with their patients. Little wonder that physicians have strong and increasing distrust of managers, politicians and governments.

The wider chaos of healthcare systems also impacts on managers. They feel bullied and scapegoated, not just by medical professionals, but also by politicians, a point that we will return to in Chapter 4. The pressures on managers can be overwhelming, with the media and politicians ever ready to condemn them for not meeting 'centrally imposed targets or face losing their jobs, while at the same time being expected to act according to longstanding principles of high public standards'.[49] Still, the feuding is always limited because the public demand that their healthcare institutions continue to serve their needs. In other words, the institutions must continue to function. Feuding has limits. Paradoxically, managers and clinicians are occasionally united in their shared suspicion of the increasing politicization of the healthcare systems like the NHS, chiefly of vote-catching plans in times of political electioneering. A rare point of agreement indeed!

---

46 Hunter 2002, p.73.
47 Ibid., p.74.
48 See Parkin 2009, p.60.
49 Greener 2009, p.242.

Model 4: Cultural splitting

The process of cultural splitting is one way for clinicians and managers to cope with these pressures. This model, with its origin in psychoanalytical thinking, is very similar to Model 3, but it contains nuances that throw further light on the division between clinicians and management.

Splitting is a psycho-cultural dynamic process whereby individuals and groups try to manage the doubts, anxieties and conflicting feelings caused by chaotic organizational cultures or just difficult work by isolating different elements of their experience to protect the apparent good from the bad.[50] This division then develops a system of relationships whereby people feel they are protected from cultural and personal collapse. The contemporary resurgence of nationalism in Western democracies, with its anti-immigrant dynamic, is an example of this splitting dynamic. Rapid social and economic changes threaten people. They want to feel good and in control of their lives again, so the more immigrants are branded as 'bad', the more the local people feel 'good'. The insight of splitting further improves the anthropological explanation of scapegoating as explained in the previous model because it introduces the pyschological insight of projection. Psychological projection is a defence mechanism whereby a person (or group) subconsciously deny their own characteristics, thoughts and feelings, which are then ascribed to others. For example, when men fail to accept their own vulnerability they can believe women are the helpless ones. When people feel threatened or inadequate they can project these negative feelings and impulses on to others as individuals or as groups. We are 'good'; they are 'bad'.

In the face of ongoing uncertainty in healthcare, the potential for dangerous splitting arises in many areas, such as between acute and community care, nurses and patients, doctors and nurses, CEO and

50   See Larry Hirschhorn and Donald R. Young (1991) 'Dealing with Anxiety of Working: Social Defenses as Coping Strategy.' In Manfred F. R. Kets de Vries and Associates (eds) *Organizations on the Couch: Clinical Perspectives on Organizational Behavior and Change.* San Francisco, CA: Jossey-Bass, pp.215–240. Psychoanalyst Melanie Klein discovered that the unconscious dynamic of splitting begins very early in life; in early infancy a child separates good and bad experiences of the same object (breast) or person (mother). Klein points out that it is a sign of maturity for a person to accept the emotions of hate and love for the same person, without escaping into the false comfort of splitting. See Melanie Klein (1955) *New Directions in Psychoanalysis.* London: Tavistock.

management, management and departments of health. Psychoanalyst Isabel Menzies Lyth, in her research study of nursing staff in British hospitals, observed how nurses were able to cope with the emotionally stressful nature of their work with patients. Sick people became the 'cancer cases in room three' (that is, the 'good' pole) rather than having to use personal names (that 'bad' pole). In this way they did not have to relate to patients as whole people.[51] The one that particularly concerns us here, however, is the potential split between doctors and management.

CASE STUDY: DOCTORS AND MANAGEMENT

Once, when consulting to a hospital, I heard staff members making derogatory comments about the accounts department. The department had been mismanaged for several years and clinical staff particularly had benefited from this. A new CEO of the hospital hired a new departmental head to reform the entire accounting system, evoking strong hostility from the staff against the entire department, with the manager and CEO, in particular, receiving the most criticism. For example, clinical staff saw themselves as 'good' and the management in general as 'bad', because they believed the latter despised them. I tried to reason with them by explaining that the reform was necessary for the sake of the entire hospital, but to no effect. As I listened I concluded that the hostility and prejudice that staff claimed the accounts department, CEO and management had against them was in fact their own. They simply projected these qualities on to the innocent members of the department.

Responses

For the sake of patient welfare and safety there must be solutions to this schism-like behaviour. As Peter Garling, inquiring into the crises within the public hospitals of New South Wales, stated: 'To start with, a new culture needs to take root which sees the patient's needs as the paramount central concern of the system and not the

---

51   Lyth 1988, pp.48–83.

convenience of the clinicians and administrators.'[52] Unless there is energetic and sustained participation in decision-making by physicians and management, finite resources will continue to be used to the disadvantage of patients and healthcare institutions. However, for a new culture to emerge, there must be clinician *and* management *leadership*, and ideally managers with clinical backgrounds. It is difficult to achieve a new culture of collaboration given the fact that there are inbuilt resistances to change in all cultures and subcultures (see Guidelines 2 and 3, Chapter 1). Everyone will give lip-service to quality and excellence in patient care, but I am advocating that professionals and managers will be required to make radical changes in attitudes and behaviour in order to work together to implement high-quality, cost-effective patient care. As already explained, physicians are highly individualistic, even when they work in small groups of four or five. To attempt to bring these groups into a larger practice entity, first to collaborate among themselves and then with management, is a monumental challenge.[53] It is difficult for clinicians to realize that 'poor management practice is as at least as lethal as poor clinical practice'.[54] The situation is made more complicated by the fact that a significant number of doctors have split loyalties – to their hospitals and to their private practices. Richard Smith, editor of the *British Medical Journal*, warned doctors that they are 'losing out in modern healthcare systems because of their discomfort with leadership, strategy, systems thinking, negotiation, genuine team working, organizational development, economics, and finance'.[55] Yet doctors and nurses can feel that time spent on management is 'time consuming, emotionally draining, and at times, nerve-racking experience. Time devoted to management activities…is inevitably in conflict with either clinical or private time.'[56] Moreover, clinical involvement in management is apt to be financially unrewarding.

---

52 Garling, 2008b, p.3

53 See Stephen M. Shortell *et al.* (2000) *Remaking Health Care in America: The Evolution of Organized Delivery Systems.* San Francisco, CA: Jossey-Bass, p.85.

54 Edwards *et al.* 2003, p.609.

55 Richard Smith (2003) 'What doctors and managers can learn from each other.' *British Medical Journal 326* (22 March), 611.

56 Jenny Simpson (1994) 'Doctors and management – why bother?' *British Medical Journal 309* (3 December), 1506.

Overall, the obstacles are so great that collaboration may seem an impossible task. However, at times it can and does happen. For example, in Britain and in the United States, it has been found 'that hospitals with the greatest clinician participation in management scored about 50% higher on important drivers of performance than hospitals with low levels of clinical leadership'.[57] In one British study, it was 'found that CEOs in the highest-performing organizations engaged clinicians in dialogue and in joint problem-solving efforts'.[58] The following examples illustrate the reasons for successful collaboration.

CASE STUDIES: CLINICIAN AND MANAGEMENT PARTNERSHIPS

New Zealand

Clinical leadership and partnership with management can be achieved, as demonstrated by the collaborative work in New Zealand. There were three contributing factors: first, the relatively low level of financial investment by government in healthcare forced clinicians and management to develop a greater degree of collaboration; second, following the revelation in 1987 that a physician had been intentionally under-treating women with cervical cancer and experimenting on his patients without their consent and proper approval,[59] the medical profession took the initiative to foster greater collective professional accountability and collaborative partnership with management; and third, the neoliberal reforms had been so devastating in the 1990s that both the medical clinicians and management recognized that they must collaborate in order to bring stability back to the public health system for the sake of patients' safety and welfare. It is significant that the initiatives for collaboration and more clinical transparency came particularly from clinical leadership, in reaction to the public exposure of poor clinical accountability and transparency.[60]

---

57   See James Mountford and Caroline Webb (2009) 'When clinicians lead.' *McKinsey Quarterly* (February), 3.

58   Ibid. The study referred to is: Academy of Royal Medical Colleges and NHS Institute (2007) *Enhancing Engagement in Medical Leadership.* Available at www.institute.nhs.uk.

59   See Cheyne *et al.* 2008, p.219.

60   See Laurence Malcolm, Lyn Wright, Pauline Barnett and Chris Hendry (2003) 'Building a successful partnership between management and clinical leadership: Experience from New Zealand.' *British Medical Journal 326* (22 March), 653–654.

USA: Kaiser Permanente

Kaiser Permanente, America's largest HMO, provoked widespread anger from the medical establishment when it introduced a system of shared 'responsibility and accountability for overall performance of health systems'. The result is 'an organisational culture that transcends the traditional conflicts between "medicine" and "management"'.[61]

Four factors have contributed to this achievement: first, and fundamental to the founding vision of the HMO, was the requirement at the highest level of the organization for partnership, which would become the model for collaboration at all levels; second, it was recognized that fundamental to the subcultures of management and clinicians were common values such as concern for patient welfare. A mutually interdependent relationship based on these values would benefit not just the patients, but all involved in the relationship. Third, appropriate leadership and management training was and continues to be provided for doctors so that 'physician leaders now understand both the bedside and the boardroom and make competent partners for similarly well trained managers'.[62] Fourth, this partnership culture did not happen overnight. Rather, it has been fostered 'over decades of continuous negotiation by hundreds of committees and leadership councils that jointly manage the organisation on a daily basis'.[63]

The lessons of these case studies are universally applicable.

Lesson 1: Shared mission and values

Commitment to a common mission and values alone will bind people together in a common task. Both subcultures must have the *same* mission and values – the safety and the quality of care of the patient,[64] but they will contribute to this end in different ways. As Huw Thomas and Stephen Pattison concluded:

> If professionals, users and institutions are to pull together with some commonality of goal, intent, ends and means, then, in one form or another, they will have to engage within the field of values...

---

61 See Francis J. Crosson (2003) 'Kaiser Permanente: A propensity for partnership.' *British Medical Journal 326* (22 March), 654.
62 Ibid.
63 Ibid.
64 See Garling, 2008b., p.7.

Failure to do this is likely to result in a frustrating dissipation of energy and good will as people work against, rather than with, each other.[65]

But the formulation of this common mission and values takes time and the temptation for members of both subcultures to give up will need to be resisted. There must be regular times set aside for clinicians and managers to develop a shared-value approach to their work. The values must be frequently and explicitly restated and their practical implications discussed in a non-blaming, non-confrontational atmosphere. This is achievable *only* with people gifted with leadership qualities, commitment to a vision and the ability to draw others into collaborative and creative strategies.

The emphasis on common values is conceptually not the same as compromise. The latter is founded on achieving equilibrium of power, but this is bound to be an unstable arrangement because power relations can alter. What is being proposed here, however, is a sharing of values which must endure and guide all decision-making throughout healthcare institutions.[66] While not denying the important contribution to the process on the part of managers, nonetheless, I agree with James Mountford and Caroline Webb that 'leadership must come substantially from doctors and other clinicians, whether or not they play formal management roles'.[67] The primary task of clinicians and healthcare services is healing. Ultimately, therefore, clinicians should hold the leadership roles, not people whose chief skills is business management. It is taken for granted that headmasters of schools and vice-chancellors of universities must be experts in education, not business management. So, also in healthcare; clinicians are the professionals in healing, not business managers.[68] However, often they lack the skills, self-confidence or language to enter into dialogue about values, but the welfare and safety of their patients demand these barriers are overcome in order

---

65   Huw Thomas and Stephen Pattison (2010) 'Health Care Professions and their Changing Values: Pulling Professions Together.' In Stephen Pattison, Ben Hannigan, Roisin Pill and Huw Thomas (eds) *Emerging Values in Health Care*. London: Jessica Kingsley Publishers, p.230.
66   See Drife and Johnston 1995, p.1056.
67   Mountford and Webb 2009, p.3.
68   See James Dunbar, Prasuna Reddy and Stephen May (2011) *Deadly Healthcare*. Bowen Hills, Queensland: Australian Academic Press, pp.154–156.

to move forward.[69] Doctors are particularly uncomfortable with discussions of abstract values, tending 'to be reactive – driven by science and suffering'.[70] Managers for their part might well learn from medical clinicians the importance of developing a stronger evidence base for their work, as well as keeping as close to patients as is possible.

Lesson 2: Government obstructive interference

Governments have a vital role in encouraging teamwork between clinicians and managers. But in countries like the United States, and now in England, where the government policy is to emphasize choice and competition, values which conflict with those of the founding mythology of healthcare, the task of fostering a common mission and values is so much more difficult. In addition to the existing distrust of managers, clinicians view managers as agents of government policies who cannot be trusted to enter into honest dialogue. As David Hunter wrote: 'The politicisation of management and the consequent distortion of the values managers might otherwise wish to uphold is a serious obstacle to achieving a set of shared values.'[71] It is not surprising, in these circumstances, that doctors see themselves as the only remaining protectors of the founding mythology.[72]

Lesson 3: Modelling

Examples of success stories, in which tribal barriers are overcome, can model for others what can be achieved through multidisciplinary teamwork.[73]

---

69   See Thomas and Pattison 2010, p.235.
70   Smith 2003, p.611.
71   Hunter 2002, p.77.
72   Ibid., pp.72–73.
73   For a review of the successes and challenges of building a multidisciplinary team of clinicians in a department of an Australian public hospital, see Debbi Long, Bonsan B. Lee and Jeffrey Braithwaite (2008) 'Attempting Clinical Democracy: Enhancing Multivocality in a Multidisciplinary Clinical Team.' In Carmen R. Cladas-Coulthard and Rick Iedema (eds) *Identity Trouble: Critical Discourse and Contested Identities.* Basingstoke: Palgrave Macmillan, pp.250–272.

Lesson 4: Education

There needs to be appropriate management and leadership formation in the undergraduate and early clinical training years.[74] It is unfortunate that leadership and management formation is still lacking from the core curricula for many undergraduate and postgraduate programmes.[75] For example, given the poverty of existing formation programmes for clinicians in management, the original proposal (now very significantly modified) of the British Government in 2010–2011 to transfer the power to commission £80 billion of care annually from PCTs to general practitioners seemed rather naive. Many general practitioners, concluded an editorial to *The Times*, 'may be unwilling to shoulder so heavy an administrative burden, with little incentive to do so beyond the altruistic. Or, indeed, they may simply be no better at it than the trusts they replace.'[76] If general practitioners are unwilling or unable, the way is wide open for for-profit administrators to enter. Then the process of privatization and corporatization could further jeopardize the founding values of solidarity, equity, justice, compassion.

Summary

○ Tribal tensions between clinicians and managers are a reality. Not only is this detrimental to patients, but it also in danger of 'alienating the most skilled in the medical workforce from service in the public system'.[77] Efforts to encourage better communication and collaboration are often weakened 'by differential power and status, lack of interprofessional socialisation, and inadequate time devoted to team building'.[78] While this chapter has concentrated on the relations between clinicians and managers, similar tensions exist between other clinicians, for example, nurses and management. Nurses are also unhappy when they are required to spend more and more

---

74 See Garling, 2008b, p.5.
75 See Mountford and Webb 2009, p.6.
76 'Editorial: Hospital pass.' (2011) *The Times* (January 17), 2.
77 Garling, 2008b, p.11.
78 Sisse Neale and Graham Neale (2005) 'Clinical leadership in the provision of hospital care.' *British Medical Journal 330* (28 May), 1219.

time on management issues since they feel this increasingly isolates them from their primary task – the care of patients.

○ Ultimately tribalism is a struggle to maintain or achieve *power*. As explained in Chapter 1 power subtly permeates every facet of a culture or subculture and can be psychologically all-encompassing and oppressive, without the people involved being aware of what is happening. This makes collaboration between members of the two subcultures difficult to achieve. The power of clinicians to influence healthcare decisions has dramatically weakened over the past 20 years. This loss of power results in behaviour that can be harmful to all concerned, especially patients. As the 2001 final report into medical malpractice of two surgeons at the Bristol Royal Infirmary concluded, 'when tribal groups fall out, or disagree over territory in an organisation such as the NHS, the safety and quality of the care given to the patient is put at risk'.[79]

○ Teamwork is generally very messy, because it is a human activity involving cultural change, and the personalities, emotions and quirks of many creative people. Yet teamwork at all levels is crucial to healthcare reform.[80] Teamwork is the result of a high level of interdependency and trust; that is, each person in the team has their role clarified and feels responsible for, and is supported in, its achievement, but at the same time is working to combine their own actions with those of others in view of *a commonly accepted mission* and values. That is, collaboration and trust across professional boundaries is possible, when those involved accept and commit themselves to a founding mythology on which a common mission and values ultimately depend. When this commitment does not exist, or breaks down, then collaboration becomes impossible. Feuding and 'tribal warfare' between the subcultures results.

79   Bristol Royal Infirmary Inquiry (2001) *Learning from Bristol: The Report of the Public Inquiry into Children's Heart Surgery at the Bristol Royal Infirmary 1984–1995*. Accessed on 12/6/12 at www. bristol-inquiry.org.uk/, p.276.
80   Thomas H. Lee concludes that the development of teams among physicians at Pennsylvania's Geisinger Health System has helped to halve hospital readmissions. See Lee 2010, p.56.

◉ Healthcare managers and clinicians need each other. Therefore, managers must foster the collaboration, especially of medical clinicians, in policy and implementation strategies. Since the 1980s, with the emphasis on corporatization in healthcare, medical clinicians have increasingly been excluded from decision-making processes, a recipe that can only lead to increased tribal tensions.

Stratetic implications
Policies

◉ Tribal-like tensions between managers and clinicians, especially medical clinicians, threaten the safety and health of patients. It is essential, therefore, that effective measures be taken to develop more constructive relationships. When senior administrators and clinicians proactively assume this responsibility, very positive results can be expected, setting an example for others in the healthcare system to follow.[81]

Implementation

◉ Because medical clinicians have in recent decades increasingly lost executive authority in hospitals, it is imperative that they again be truly involved in decision-making in matters that pertain to their expertise. Incidents of successful collaboration among clinicians and between clinicians and managers need to be published in order to encourage others to follow their example.[82]

◉ One way to foster collaboration and mutual trust is to develop multidisciplinary ward visits to patients; this provides opportunities for clinicians such as physicians, nurses and allied staff to share expert information and come to know one another better on a personal and professional level.

---

81   See NSW Independent Panel (2010a) *Independent Panel: Caring Together: The Health Action Plan for NSW: Second Progress Report (June 2010)*. Sydney: NSW Independent Panel, p.37.
82   Ibid.

○ Since full clinical engagement in decision-making will not occur if senior medical clinicians are not prepared to lead, everything possible needs to be done to encourage individuals to become role models for others.

○ Managers should insist that part-time medical clinicians fulfil their contractual, collaborative obligations to hospitals; failure to do so weakens the credibility of the managers and undermines efforts to achieve wider collaboration among clinicians and others.

○ Because culture shock is more likely to happen when managers and clinicians are insensitive to cultural differences between them, it is imperative that in their initial and ongoing training they develop attitudes and skills of communication that understand and respect cultural diversity; this will discourage harmful tribal-like behaviours between the two subcultures.[83]

---

83   See Gary L. Kreps and Elizabeth N. Kunimoto (1994) *Effective Communication in Multicultural Health Care Settings*. Thousand Oaks, CA: Sage Publications, p.24.

CHAPTER 4

Bullying in Healthcare Institutions

An Anthropological Perspective

Bullying renders the victim impotent: fear paralyses.
(Ruth Hadikin)[1]

This chapter explains:

○ the meaning of bullying and harassment behaviour and its prevalence in healthcare cultures

○ that this behaviour takes many different forms that can be summarized under the titles of persistent critic, skilled manipulator, space invader, benevolent intimidator and irresponsible abdicator

○ that particular culture models encourage bullying: resource-limited, hierarchical, win–lose, envy/jealousy and political 'cargo cult'

○ that the values-based model focuses on building a culture of justice.

Bullying is not confined to children. It is, in fact, a widespread form of abuse to be found in all forms of employment, cultures, politics and churches.[2] When it is encouraged in healthcare cultures, staff experience unnecessary stress and loss of energy and move to more

---

1   Ruth Hadikin and Muriel O'Driscoll (2000) *The Bullying Culture.* Oxford: Butterworth-Heinemann, p.75; this quote is reproduced with the permission of Elsevier.

2   See Peter Randall's analysis regarding statistics of bullying: (2001) *Bullying in Adulthood: Assessing the Bullies and their Victims.* Hove: Routledge, pp.7–18.

harmonious workplaces. Patient care and safety are jeopardized.[3] It is estimated that one-third to one-half of all stress-related sicknesses in Western countries result from workplace bullying. The personal consequences of bullying can be disastrous: depression, memory loss and feelings of hopelessness, even post-traumatic stress disorder.[4] Moreover, bullying strikes at the fundamental values of solidarity, respect, compassion and justice that lie at the heart of the founding story of healthcare (see Chapter 2). The purpose of this chapter is to identify the cultures that readily foster this significant problem in healthcare systems.

A nationwide study of staff in the British NHS concluded that three in five people had witnessed bullying at their work in the previous two years.[5] According to a 2008 government report, nearly 1 in 12 staff working in the NHS had experienced bullying or harassment by their manager.[6] One Australian survey discovered that over 50 per cent of Australian junior doctors had been bullied by senior clinicians in their workplace, and a New Zealand survey concluded that 50 per cent of doctors had experienced at least one incident of bullying during their previous three- or six-month clinical attachment.[7] Often healthcare systems have extensive policies and guidelines to prevent bullying, but they prove to be ineffective.[8] The human and financial

---

3   Rhona Flin, Professor of Applied Psychology, University of Aberdeen, notes that studies suggest 'that in confined work areas, such as operating theatres, even watching rudeness that occurs colleagues might impair team members' thinking skills… [The] risks for surgical patients – whose treatment depends on particularly high levels of mental concentration and flawless task execution – could increase.' Rhona Flin (2010) 'Rudeness at work: A threat to patient safety and quality of care.' *British Medical Journal 341* (31 July), 212–213. Rudeness can be a form of bullying.

4   See David Kinchin (1998) *Post-Traumatic Stress Disorder: The Invisible Injury.* London: Success Unlimited.

5   See UNISON (2003) *Bullying at Work.* London: UNISON, p.5. Accessed 15 June 2012 at www.unison.org.uk/acrobat/13375.pdf; also Cheryl Hume, Jacqueline Randle and Keith Stevenson (2006) 'Student Nurses' Experience of Workplace Relationships.' In Jacqueline Randle (ed.) *Workplace Bullying in NHS.* Oxford: Radcliffe, pp.63–74. See also Lyne Quine (1999) 'Workplace bullying in NHS Community Trust: Staff questionnaire survey.' *British Medical Journal 318* (23 January), 228–232.

6   Jo Revill (2008) 'NHS bosses "bully one in 12 staff."' *Observer* (27 January). Accessed 15 June 2012 at www.guardian.co.uk/society/2008/jan/27/nhs.bullying.

7   See Joanne Scott, Chloe Blanshard and Stephen Child (2008) 'Workplace bullying of junior doctors: A cross sectional questionnaire survey.' *New Zealand Medical Journal Digest 121*, 1282, 13–15.

8   See Garling 2008a, pp.399–425.

costs of bullying are enormous.[9] When the perpetrators are medical clinicians, especially if they bring in significant revenue to hospitals and/or if they are owners of the facilities, administrators hesitate to challenge their dysfunctional behaviour. Workplace bullying in healthcare facilities encourages medical mistakes, is a factor in poor patient satisfaction, disrupts teamwork, creates low staff morale, causes absenteeism and ill-health in victims, and encourages staff, including qualified clinical and administrative staff members, to move to safer and more supportive professional positions elsewhere.[10] In the United States, a 2008 study of medical malpractice cases found that these frequently resulted from poor communication between staff members; a prominent cause of communication was workplace bullying.[11] In an earlier study (2004), 49 per cent of healthcare professionals reported that bullying negatively affected the way they dealt with questions concerning medication orders.[12]

Defining bullying and harassment

We need to be quite clear what bullying means. It is often used loosely to describe any stressful interaction between peers or between employees and employers. Employers have the right and duty to call staff members to account, but to do this in a firm but respectful manner. Employees may find this stressful, but it is not bullying.[13]

9 According to one estimate published in 2009, workplace bullying and harassment cost the NHS more than £325 million annually. See Rachael Heenan (2009) 'How to beat NHS workplace bullying.' *HSJ* (9 Febraury), 1. Accessed 5 April 2010 at www.hsj.co.uk/new/workforce/how-to-beat-nhs-workplace-bullying/1970330 article.

10 See the Joint Commission on Accreditation of Healthcare organization, (JCAHO) (2008) 'Sentinel event alter: Behaviors that undermine a culture of safety.' Accessed 5/4/10 at www.jointcommission.org/assets/1/18/SEA_40.pdf.

11 Ibid.

12 See Institute for Safe Medical Practices (ISMP) (2004) 'Intimidation: Practitioners speak up about this unresolved problem (Part 1)' Accessed 14 April 2011 at https://ismp.org/Newsletters/acutecare/articles/20040311_2.asp.

13 See Frank Furedi (1998) *Culture of Fear: Risk-taking and the Morality of Low Expectation.* London: Cassell, pp.73–105.

DEFINITION

Bullying is an act of violence involving the abuse of power by individuals, groups, institutions or cultures, so that individuals or groups not in a position to defend themselves are downgraded as human persons through being persistently subjected to threats of psychological, physical or cultural violence, which weakens their self-confidence and self-esteem, so facilitating their subjugation.[14] The term 'harassment' is used to describe a specific form of bullying in which the victim belongs to a legally protected group such as race, sex, sexual orientation or disability.

The key terms in this definition are *act of violence, abuse of power* and that which *weakens their self-confidence and self-esteem, so facilitating their subjugation.*

Violence

Bullying is an act of violence. Commonly, violence is defined as the infliction of physical harm to the human body or to human property through the use of either the body or weapons. Such a description is too restrictive: it would confine bullying to the application of physical force. A preferable definition, therefore, stresses violence as the 'exercise of physical or emotional force to injure or abuse someone'.[15] Even this preferred definition needs to be expanded, however, to include cultural or structural violence.

14 See Gerald A. Arbuckle (2003) *Dealing with Bullies.* London: St Pauls Publishing, pp.17–25.
15 Gerard Vanderhaar (1998) *Beyond Violence.* Mystic, CT: Twenty-Third Publications, p.32.

VIOLENCE: BACKGROUND

Social scientists and philosophers have disagreed for centuries over whether aggression (which lies behind violence) is innate or instinctive or learned. The philosopher Thomas Hobbes (1588–1679) believed that individuals have no altruistic tendency nor any natural inclination towards mutual help or peaceful life with others: people act like wolves to obtain what they want. Similarly, Friedrich Nietzsche (1844–1900) claimed that the inner drive for personal advantage favours violence. The psychoanalyst Sigmund Freud (1856–1939) concluded that aggression is a consequence of the human death drive. When this instinct is turned inwards, the death wish shows itself in self-punishment which, in extreme situations, leads to suicide. Erich Fromm (1900–1980) claimed that violence is due to the constrictions of civilized society. For Melanie Klein (1882–1960), a psychoanalyst, violence is instinctual and inborn; violators project their own inner fears and inadequacies on to other people and society. Bullies are inadequate people, fearful of losing face, overly sensitive to criticism, deeply lonely within themselves. According to Klein, bullies experience an inner fury over their personal failures and project them on to some other object, in this case, the victim. The victim chosen as the target of the inner rage becomes the 'bad object' to be crushed. Klein argued: 'Original aggression is expelled as a danger and established elsewhere as something bad, and then the object invested with dangerousness becomes a target at which aggression arising subsequently can be discharged.'[20] The 'bad object', the victim, can then be freely ill treated and its destruction becomes acceptable.

Psychologists generally identify two major conditions that can provoke an individual to violence: first, frustration resulting from failure to achieve one's desires; and, second, an attack or threat of attack on one's life, material well-being, self-image or

---

16   Melanie Klein and Joan Riviere (1964) *Love, Hate and Reparation.* New York: Norton, p.13.

self-esteem.[17] Psychologists write a great deal on violence, detailing the psychological inadequacies of perpetrators and the effects on the victim.[18] However, social psychologists, who are primarily concerned about the ways in which individual behaviour is affected by the lives of others, commonly accept that the causes of violence are deeply rooted in human nature *and* culture. For a social psychologist violence may be a way to avoid boredom, to raise self-esteem in the presence of others, to express frustration at not getting what one wants or to achieve status in society.

Social anthropology's contribution to our understanding of violence through bullying, by contrast, is twofold: first, it highlights cultural and historical pressures which have strong and unappreciated roles that contribute to violence; and second, it examines social realities in a cross-cultural frame of reference. For the anthropologist, violence is pre-eminently collective rather than individual, usually culturally structured and always culturally interpreted. The main emphasis in this chapter, therefore, is to focus not on individual bullying as violent behaviour, but on identifying entrenched processes in cultures that foster or allow violence to occur.[19] It is argued that a culture of bullying or abuse is a collection of traditions, conventions and language that can be used within a group to legitimize mistreatment of its members or of outsiders. Unless cultures are examined and modified, the intimidation of the powerless will continue.

Abuse of power

Peter Randall, a British authority on workplace bullying, commented: 'It is axiomatic that wherever there is power, it is likely to be abused, and wherever there is vulnerability there is likely to be exploitation.'[20] In the hospital system the bully places their personal agenda of controlling another person above the needs of patients and staff members. Employees everywhere have a right to feel both

---

17   See Ervin Staub (1989) *The Roots of Evil: The Origins of Genocide and Other Group Violence.* Cambridge: Cambridge University Press, p.35.

18   For example, see Andrea Adams (1992) *Bullying at Work.* London: Virago Press; Gary Namie and Ruth Namie (2000) *The Bully at Work.* Naperville, IL: Sourcebooks; Ken Rigby (2002) *New Perspectives on Bullying.* London: Jessica Kingsley Publishers.

19   See Hadikin and O'Driscoll 2000.

20   Peter Randall (1997) *Adult Bullying: Perpetrators and Victims.* London: Routledge, p.49.

physically and psychologically safe in their workplace,[21] especially in healthcare institutions committed to healing. The fact that bullies may be unaware of what they are doing is not the issue. If they are behaving in a bullying way, it is bullying. A physician who, without sufficient reason, consistently arrives late for procedures is acting as a bully. So also, a clinician who writes ward notes illegibly and does nothing about it is a bully. A manager who refuses to consult with medical staff before making decisions that affect them is a bully. Because employers are frequently more fearful of the workplace bully than of the victim, they dodge calling the bully to account, even if this means promoting them.[22] Patients and/or their families are known to abuse staff members. A 2006 study of healthcare workers in Britain found that 12 per cent had experienced physical violence from patients or their relatives; 26 per cent reported bullying from patients or patients' relatives.[23] However, in the absence of further reliable empirical studies it is difficult to know how widespread this problem is in other countries.

One form of abuse is the prejudicial treatment of patients on the basis of age, sex or race. For example, Augustus White of the Harvard University Medical School describes studies in the United States that illustrate how the race and sex of patients can negatively influence physicians' decisions about whether to refer for catheterization. Black or female patients were less likely to be referred for catheterization than white or male patients. Physicians may be unaware of their prejudices, but their actions are still an abuse of power and a form of bullying.[24]

Subjugation

Bullies aim to coerce people to do what they want them to do. The impact on victims can be devastating. The words of the psalmist resonate with all victims down through the centuries, as he describes his suffering as a consequence of bullying: 'Insults have broken my

21   Ibid., pp.106–117.
22   See Andrea W. Needham (2003) *Workplace Bullying: The Costly Secret*. London: Penguin, p.71.
23   Reported by Veloshnee Gvender and Loveday Penn-Kekana (2007) 'Gender Biases and Discrimination.' Geneva: World Health Organization. Accessed 25 August 2011 at www.who.int/gender_biases_and_discrimination_wgkn_2007.pdf.
24   See Augustus A. White (2011) *Seeing Patients: Unconscious Bias in Health Care*. Cambridge, MA: Harvard University Press, pp.233–255.

heart, so that I am in despair...' (Ps 69:20), 'I am utterly spent and crushed; I groan because of the tumult of my heart...' (Ps 38:8), 'I have become like a broken vessel...' (Ps 31:12). The consequence of this abuse is that the victim's self-esteem and confidence are apt to disintegrate. Bullies will use all kinds of intimidation to achieve this purpose: manipulation, abusive language, passive aggression, physical threats, public or private humiliation, refusal to take the blame for failures, trivial fault-finding, constantly being critical and sarcastic with others, withholding information to maintain power over people, scapegoating, expecting unreasonable results from others, manipulating employers against employees, refusal to delegate authority and undermining teamwork. They seek to dominate their victims for their own gratification and consequently destroy the victim's sense of self-worth. We need to remember that the contemporary bully's behaviour is *not necessarily brutish* or physically threatening. For example, bullies can be charming, sensitive, even empathetic, but their behaviour is entirely a means of maintaining their hold over others. A bully can be so successful in subjugating their victim, by using the most charming and insidious methods, that the latter comes to believe that they themselves are at fault for the violence and/or they are inferior to the perpetrator. I agree with Peter Randall that many adult bullies have Machiavellian talents in finding 'devious ways of bringing pain to their victims without discredit to themselves'.[25]

Types of bullies

While many different types of bullies may be encountered in a variety of settings, perhaps the types most often to be found in the workplace are the *persistent critic*, the *skilled manipulator*, the *space invader*, the *benevolent intimidator* and the *irresponsible abdicator*.[26]

Persistent critic

This bully subjects a victim to constant nitpicking or fault-finding, sarcastic remarks, excessive work demands, passive aggression or excessive numbers of memos or letters. The victim can feel haunted,

25   Randall 2001, p.7.
26   See Arbuckle 2003, pp.25–32.

excessively controlled and not trusted. The perpetrator can choose the most inappropriate time, for example as the victim is about to go on annual leave, to demand unreasonable reports. The following is a composite, not a specific, case study, that is, I have brought together experiences of many people I have listened to over the years describing what it meant to be bullied. So often experiences were the same.

CASE STUDY: PERSISTENT CRITIC

When the new manager of our section in the hospital assumed office, she began to write to me frequently about trivial issues and to request immediate responses. She would choose the most inappropriate times to do this, for example, just before my holidays or on the eve of presenting major reports to local government. I began to feel as though I was under a waterfall and could not escape. I felt I was constantly haunted by the leader; my sleep was affected, my energy for work declined. I just loathed going to work. No sooner had I replied to one email explaining a point than another would come demanding more information. For a while she used to phone to pressure me with questions, but eventually I was able to stop this.

In my annual reports I would explain not only what was happening in our project, but also the philosophy and values upon which it was based. The manager, however, would bypass the substance of the reports and question me about irrelevant details. Then I discovered that she had gone to the CEO in an effort to have the project put directly under her control. The CEO, after consultation with my colleagues and me, refused.

At the times when I did speak with the manager, I found myself becoming angry and weary because she would never allow me to discuss the values of the project and how the project was responding to real needs. She would become obstinate and dogmatic about little things the more I invited her to look at the bigger issues affecting the project, but she kept saying I should improve my 'public relations' with herself and the hospital, yet the more I tried the more she would interfere. It became a hopeless situation. When I tried to communicate my worries to one of her immediate advisers, I was rebuffed. The manager had sent instructions to all her advisers that their role was to support her and not to listen to complaints from staff. They were told that I was disloyal and would not listen to sound advice. I began to feel a non-person. No one in authority would listen to me.

Some staff members submitted themselves and their projects to the manager's direct control for the sake of peace, but they were enraged at having done so. On my part, I believe in my work and inwardly refuse to be demeaned. I have begun to own my own authority and, consequently, I feel better in myself. My energy is no longer being drained away by the persistent bullying.

Skilled manipulator

This bully will sulk when they cannot get their way, flatter superiors while gossiping negatively about their subordinates to them, compliment their victims one minute and berate them the next or use lies or half-truths against them. The manipulator is also adept at causing divisions in a group by cultivating favourites and marginalizing others.

Space invader

This type of bully breaches boundaries, whether they be physical, role-related or emotional. *Physical* invasion may take the form of entering the geographic or intimate territory of another person without just reason or their permission, for example, entering another's office, opening their mail and accessing their private files and computer information. One victim described what he felt in such a situation when he discovered that the private notes and research files in his office had been opened and transferred to another office without his knowledge and permission: 'I felt personally violated because the room and the files were an extension of myself. My private space had been attacked. Because no one came to my defence, I felt as though I had become a non-person socially, that I had ceased to exist.'

A bully breaches *role* boundaries when, for example, they indiscriminately withdraw authority from others or constantly interfere unnecessarily in their victim's work. *Emotional* invasion occurs when abusive language, gestures or even refusal to talk are used.

Benevolent intimidator

This bully can be skilled at hiding abusive activity. For example, it could happen that a manager decides, with the approval of his superiors, to hire several people to be his assistants, claiming that they had the right qualities. He bypasses the normal procedure whereby all positions should be advertised and applicants objectively assessed according to set criteria. But such an approach always has significant dangers. The new employees would have to feel grateful to the manager for their jobs; this could lead to a false loyalty to him and make it difficult for them to challenge his plans and behaviour. In being dependent on the manager, and so not being free to question his policies and management style, these assistants could be subjected to a subtle form of bullying by the manager.

Irresponsible abdicator

If boards of healthcare institutions fail to govern responsibly they act in a bullying manner towards innocent people, at least indirectly. For example, when CEOs, managers and supervisors fail, through neglect, to call people to be accountable for their actions, they are indirectly acting as bullies of those innocent people who suffer in consequence of this failure. Also, when board members abdicate their authority, they are power abusers and, therefore, bullies. Reflecting on his experience in the United States, William George, an expert in corporate governance, believes there is a breakdown in the principles of governance. He concluded that some boards are too smug, failing to call management to be accountable for their actions. As he writes, they do not 'challenge management… Some boards don't have the will – or the courage – to challenge a powerful CEO…Too many CEOs use their boards as a rubber stamp and actively discourage input or challenges from their independent directors.'[27]

Cultures promoting bullying: Models

Cultures subtly condition how we feel, think and act. The influence of cultures on bullying is so powerful that we can rightly speak at times

---

27   William W. George (2002) 'Imbalance of power.' *Harvard Business Review 80*, 7, 22.

of cultures of bullying. That is, cultures that allow, even encourage, people to bully others. Peter Garling, in his analysis of the workplace culture of public hospitals in New South Wales, Australia, concluded that it is 'characterised by lack of respect and trust, absence of empathy and compassion, inability to celebrate the success of others, failure to communicate, and a lack of collaboration'. No wonder, he comments, that staff feel bullied, 'victimised and powerless'.[28] When we refer to cultures of bullying in healthcare, we do not confine our comments to hospitals. Such cultures can exist also in departments of health, parliamentary departments such as those of ministers of health, even of prime ministers.

I now briefly analyse seven models of cultures of bullying: the resource-limited, hierarchical, accountability failure, win/lose, envy/jealousy, blaming and 'cargo cult' models. These oppressive models will then be contrasted with the positive values-based model. In practice, it is possible that a culture that encourages bullying will have elements of all these models, although one model will tend to be dominant at a particular time.

Model 1: Resource-limited culture

Hospitals often function in a resource-limited and highly pressurized environment – an atmosphere that is extremely conducive to dysfunctional behaviour. Working under such pressures can cause hospital staff to deal with each other and patients abruptly and abusively, so bullying increases. For example, the inquiry into the state of the Mid Staffordshire NHS Foundation Trust Hospital in 2010, where between 400 and 1200 or more patients may have died due to appalling care, found that patients were routinely neglected and left humiliated by staff. Shortages of staff caused patients to be left unwashed for weeks, without food and drink; some were left in soiled sheets that relatives had to take and wash; others developed infections or had falls, which were at times fatal.[29]

28 Garling 2008a, p.416.
29 See Francis 2010.

Model 2: Hierarchical culture

Healthcare institutions approximate to the *strong group / strong grid* culture model, as explained in Chapter 1 (see Guideline 3). In this hierarchical culture model, the boundaries of the group and the style of interpersonal relationships within it are sharply defined. People are expected to fit into a tradition-based, hierarchical system in which superiors are presumed to have a monopoly over knowledge by right of their position. There is little or no consultation in decision-making. Instead, superiors expect commands to be obeyed without question. Leaders are assumed to be stereotypically masculine, rational rather than intuitive, with an aggressive ability to command and enforce conformity. Female leaders are expected to adopt these qualities. There is considerable potential for two types of bullying in hierarchical cultures, which I term 'top-down' and 'bottom-up'.

'Top-down' bullying

In 'top-down' bullying, superiors can act with little or no organizational restraints or accountability.[30] Because they are able to control the avenues of communication, it is possible for them to conceal any abusive action.[31] Trust within the culture disintegrates. Members who have complaints become cynical about ever being listened to impartially.[32] Such was the case, for example, in the Mid Staffordshire NHS Trust, where staff members felt bullied by the board because it failed to listen to their complaints. Robert Francis, the chairman of the inquiry, concluded that the Trust's board relied too heavily on external favourable assessments, failing to take account of internal evaluations and the comments of staff and patients. On the other hand, staff members were often hesitant to complain because of perceived bullying by management.[33] This points to an in-built danger in hierarchical cultural systems. Given

30 See Angela Ishmael (1999) *Harassment, Bullying and Violence at Work.* London: Industrial Society, pp.131–132.
31 See John A. Bargh and Jeannette Alvarez (2001) 'The Road to Hell: Good Intentions in the Face of Unconscious Tendencies to Misuse Power.' In Annette Y. Lee-Chai and John A. Bargh (eds) *The Use and Abuse of Power.* New York: New York University Press, pp.41–53.
32 See Andrew J. Goldsmith (2000) 'An Impotent Conceit: Law, Culture and the Regulation of Police Violence.' In Tony Coady *et al.* (eds) *Violence and Police Culture.* Melbourne: Melbourne University Press, pp.123–125.
33 See Francis 2010, pp.152–184.

that loyalty is the pre-eminent virtue in hierarchical cultures, people daring to break the code of silence are in danger of condemnation or automatic expulsion. All kinds of negative expressions are used to describe their behaviour. They are branded and diminished with such 'dishonourable' titles as 'rats', 'squealers', 'stirrers', 'rebels', 'deviants', 'traitors to tradition'[34] and, very commonly, 'whistleblowers'.[35] The idiom 'whistleblower', however, is too weak to describe either the agonies behind this form of identifying and reporting the wrongdoing of others or its dramatic consequences. Sometimes, in hierarchical organizations, it can happen that bullies are tolerated by superiors simply because they meet targets and are financially successful. A blind eye can be turned to abusive behaviour for fear that the bullies will leave if confronted with their actions. For this reason, the superiors themselves indirectly became bullies. Better to sacrifice 'dangerous agitators' complaining about the bullying than not to achieve financial targets!

Medical clinicians are not immune from this social disease of bullying. The failure to respect sufficiently the professional qualifications of other professions, such as nurses, is a form of cultural bullying.[36] As in all professional groups, the coercive pressure to maintain silence when colleagues act incompetently is considerable. Junior doctors fear to challenge their seniors. Moreover, doctors rarely publicize bullying and malpractice of colleagues, even though the frequency of the latter indicates it must come to their notice.[37]

Bullying in healthcare also mirrors the great divide between clinicians and management. Prior to the introduction of the business model into healthcare doctors' first loyalty was to their patients. They felt morally bound to speak out when patients' rights to care

34 See Myron P. Glazer (1996) 'Ten Whistleblowers.' In M. David Erman and Richard J. Lundman (eds) *Corporate and Governmental Deviance*. New York: Oxford University Press, pp.257–277.

35 For an example see Janet B.L. Chan (1997) *Changing Police Culture: Policing in a Multicultural Society*. Cambridge: Cambridge University Press, p.80. Alexander Dyck, Adair Morse and Luigi Zingales studied 216 grave cases of fraud in US companies from 1996 to 2004. They found that four-fifths of those who revealed frauds were forced either to leave the companies, or they were fired or demoted. Their research is summarized in Tim Hartford (2011) *Adapt: Why Success Always Starts with Failure*. New York: Farrar, Strauss and Giroux, pp.210–214.

36 See Garling 2008b, p.22.

37 See conclusions by Giena Porto and Richard Lauve (2006) 'Disruptive behavior: A persistent threat to patient safety.' *Patient Safety and Quality Healthcare*. Accessed 6/8/10 at www.psqh.com/julaug06/disruptive.html.

and safety were being infringed. But with the business model in place clinicians are expected 'to put institutional loyalty before their professional values'.[38] One doctor, reflecting on his experience of a hospital culture in Sydney, Australia, complained that: 'We live in a micromanaged hell... It is run with a top-down culture of bullying and with the bottom-up response of fear and loathing.'[39] A British Medical Association survey 2009 revealed the dangers to their employment for hospital doctors who raised their concerns about the poor treatment of patients. A significant 15.5 per cent had been told by their trusts that their employment would be adversely affected if they dared to be whistleblowers.[40]

In bureaucratic health systems, like the NHS, the bullying can begin directly with politicians. Politicians, with an eye to votes, may demand, in a threatening manner, immediate answers to well-publicized problems from their health department heads, who, in turn, order in a similar way quick responses from particular managers. And so it goes down the line. For example, the insistence that national targets be met at Mid Staffordshire NHS Foundation Trust between 2005 and 2009 was described as the major reason for the shocking standards of care, particularly for patients who were admitted as emergencies and suffered unexplained high mortality rates. The demands from the Trust's board for impossible targets to be met placed intolerable burdens on understaffed facilities.[41] The insistence that unattainable targets be met started first with 'the Department of Health,'[42] no doubt under pressure from politicians. Staff struggled to comply, fearing that if targets were not achieved, their jobs would be terminated.

---

38   See Pollock 2005, p.213.
39   Quoted in Garling 2008a, p.402.
40   See British Medical Association (BMA) (2009),' 'Whisteblowing: Advice for BMA Members Working in NHS Secondary Care about Raising Concerns in the Workplace.' p.12. Accessed on 3 March 2010 at www.bma.org.uk/m/media/files/pdfs/Whistleblowing.ashx; also see Jonathan Gornall (2009) 'The price of silence.' *British Medical Journal 339* (31 October), 1000–1004, and Nina Lakhani (2009) 'NHS is paying millions to gag whistleblowers.' *Independent* (1 November), 1–10. Accessed on 4 March 2010 at www.independent.co.uk/nhs-is-paying-millions-to-gay-whistleblo. Richard Smith, editor of the *British Medical Journal* in 1994, wrote in an article 'The rise of Stalinism in the NHS' that senior staff 'were convinced that the NHS was becoming an organization in which people were terrified to speak the truth', (1994) *British Medical Journal 309* (17 December), 1640.
41   See Francis 2010, pp.151–182.
42   Ibid., p.162.

It can be perplexing to discover that people, while expressing significant satisfaction with their workplace culture, at the same time record examples of bullying either personally or by others. While there may be many reasons for this apparently contradictory experience, there is a possible anthropological explanation. As earlier explained in Chapter 1, every culture is not an entity or a material object, but a struggling process made up of numerous interacting, conflicting and dividing subcultures, their borders permeable.[43] Thus a hospital culture is not one large static entity unit, with all its constituent parts ultimately functioning systematically to produce an orderly, well-bounded whole. On the contrary, it is more akin to a chaotic process involving multiple subcultures, with changing boundaries that are sometimes overlapping, sometimes separating, sometimes in conflict, as the struggle for power and limited resources continues. A doctor, for example, may in the course of one day shift from a theatre subculture to a ward subculture, from a classroom to an administrative office. This occurs similarly with other staff members. At a particular time, one subculture will be more important for the person or the group than the others in determining their experience. This constant shifting across boundaries can be termed 'situational identity', that is, a person's or group's experience will depend on the subcultural context in which they find themselves at a particular moment and place.[44] It is thus possible for a person to be the target of personal bullying, or to observe others as victims, in a particular subculture, but be very satisfied with their workplace experience in another subculture. The satisfaction experienced in one or more subcultures outweighs for the moment the negative encounters with bullying in other subcultural contexts.

'Bottom-up' bullying

Bottom-up bullying occurs when staff collectively, and without justification, express their dislike of superiors. This usually takes the form of passive aggressive behaviour. Their dislike is fuelled by gossip, that is, the intimate exchange of prejudicial information about

---

43   See Alan Barnard (2000) *History and Theory in Anthropology*. Cambridge: Cambridge University Press, pp.158–184; Arbuckle 2010, pp.5–18.
44   See Arbuckle 2004, pp.27–28.

people who normally are not present. Gossip is about clarifying social boundaries. It is a process of including or excluding people from social relations and identification with a particular group.[45] The process of exclusion is commonly an act of silent violence toward those who are the targets of the gossip. For example, in healthcare institutions bottom-up bullying can occur if clinicians as a group blindly refuse to accept that their managers ever act in good faith. Gossip can be a relatively secure method of power manipulation for those who foster it for two reasons: first, the gossiper asserts to be just passing on information and denies any responsibility for its truthfulness; and second, it is also done under a cloak of secrecy. Sociologist Samuel Heilman referred to gossip as 'surreptitious aggression, which enables one to wrest power, manipulate, and strike out at another without the other being able to strike back'.[46]

Model 3: Accountability failure culture

This model exists when staff members are not regularly called to be accountable for their behaviour. The culture tolerates failures, with, at times, enormous costs to patients who often suffer in consequence. In the United States, for example, it has been estimated that about 4000 wrong-side surgeries are performed annually. Most could be prevented if physicians were called to be accountable to established protocols. Moreover, it is also thought that 'many, if not most, of the estimated 100,000 annual deaths from health care-associated infections in the United States could be prevented by strict adherence to infection-control practices, including hand hygiene.'[47] Peter Garling reported of public hospitals in New South Wales that a 'sizeable proportion of [clinicians who] trail infection around like sparks in a dry wheat field…bring great risk to the patients' simply

---

45 Ibid., pp.75–100; Max Gluckman (1963) 'Gossip and scandal.' *Current Anthropology 4*, 4, 309.

46 Samuel Heilman, cited by Patricia Spacks (1986) *Gossip*. Chicago, IL: University of Chicago Press, p.30.

47 Robert M. Watcher and Peter J. Pronovost (2009) 'Balancing "no blame" with accountability in patient safety.' *New England Journal of Medicine 361*, 14, 1402; see also Donald Goldman (2006) 'System failure versus personal accountability – the case for clean hands.' *New England Journal of Medicine 355*, 2, 121–123.

because they largely 'do not practise hand hygiene before and after seeing each patient'.[48]

Model 4: Win/lose culture

In the win/lose culture model, people are individualistic, utilitarian and competitive, but have a very weak sense of belonging or of having obligations to the group or institution. Individuals form alliances with one another to provide better opportunities for personal success, but these break apart once more strategically profitable relationships develop. Egotism and unrestrained, aggressive competitiveness set the scene for a culture in which people and institutions are encouraged to bully one another for their own personal advantage.

This culture model flourishes in contemporary political and business circles under the influence of neoliberalist or economic rationalist philosophy.[49] Among the things that economic rationalism fosters is a culture of sacrifice in which excessive work is forced on employees.[50] Midwives, for example, have been unduly pressured to accept excessive workloads in an Australian hospital. They feared retribution if they complained.[51] Also, when governments and supporters of neoliberal economics blame people who are poor for their own poverty, disabilities and ill health, they deprive them of necessary welfare assistance. This is an example of win/lose cultural bullying. Such is the case in the United States, for example, whenever injudicious cuts are made to welfare, unemployment benefits, Medicare and Medicaid.[52] Sociologist Robert Alford, reflecting on the American scene in 1980, was able to identify a new and emerging group of people in healthcare services who had become devotees of the economic rationalist philosophy. He called them the 'corporate rationalizers',[53] and they were to be found among

---

48   Garling 2008b, p.16.

49   See John R. Saul (1992) *Voltaire's Bastards: The Dictatorship of Reason in the West*. London: Penguin, p.106.

50   See John Wright (2003) *The Ethics of Economic Rationalism*. Sydney: University of New South Wales Press, pp.vi–viii.

51   See Garling 2008a, p.406.

52   Peter Saunders (2002) *The Ends and Means of Welfare: Coping with Economic and Social Change in Australia*. Cambridge: Cambridge University Press, p.250.

53   For an overview of the impact of economic rationalism on healthcare in United States, see Vicento Navarro (1994) *The Politics of Health Policy: The US Reforms 1980–1994*. Oxford: Blackwell.

hospital administrators, hospital insurance executives, corporate executives and bankers, medical school directors, and city and state public health administrators. Thirty years later, the situation has not changed. In England, whenever governments consistently ignore the widening gap between the rich and poor, between social classes, between north and south, and between the inner city and shire counties, they are perpetuating a win/lose culture of bullying. With poverty goes poor health. The Marmot Review on health inequalities in England in 2010 concluded that many people could not believe that serious health inequalities exist in England, but the fact is that 'in the wealthiest part of London...a man can expect to live to 88 years, while a few kilometres away...in one of the capital's poorer wards, male life expectancy is 71'.[54] The Marmot Review concluded with this condemnation of the win/lose economic philosophy, drawing readers back to the central value of social justice in the original founding of the NHS: 'The central tenet of this Review is that avoidable health inequalities are unfair and putting them right is a matter of social justice.'[55]

The biomedical model of healthcare, particularly favoured by economic rationalists, also contributes to the culture of bullying in which the poor are the victims; members of the medical profession must bear some responsibility for this. Historically the medical profession has been less concerned with social reform, public hygiene, sanitation and community services than with fostering medical technology and healing rooted in exact scientific laboratory processes. The health of a society is wrongly assumed to be mainly dependent on the state of medical expertise and the availability of medical resources. Hence, hospital-based, high technology medicine continues to receive the greatest share of healthcare budgets, all with the strong support of the middle and upper socioeconomic population. Today, as noted earlier, 'only 4 per cent of NHS funding is spent on prevention'.[56] The poor suffer the most from this over-emphasis on identification of healthcare with hospital services; hospitals, with their emphasis on the biomedical model, cannot alone achieve equality of healthcare. The social model of health, by

---

54   Marmot Review 2010, p.29.
55   Ibid.
56   Ibid., p.28.

contrast, assumes that the patterns of health and disease are largely the product of economic and cultural influences such as poverty, pollution, unemployment, racism and social discrimination.[57]

Model 5: Envy/jealousy culture

O, beware, my Lord, of jealousy!
It is the green-ey'd monster, which doth mock
The meat it feeds on.

(William Shakespeare)[58]

The report on the workplace culture of public hospitals of New South Wales noted that there is 'an inability to celebrate the success of others'.[59] This is a polite way of saying that the vices of envy and jealousy are significantly evident in the culture.[60] Envy and jealousy are almost taboo subjects in conversation and literature, even though they have bedevilled humankind from the beginning.[61] Even social scientists have been hesitant to write about them, possibly because they are such unpalatable topics for writers and readers.[62] Yet envy and jealousy are commonly causes of the misuse of power in gossip, scapegoating and bullying. It is important to recognize the similarities and differences in these two words – envy and jealousy. Envy is the sadness a person or group feels because of what someone else has and the desire or wish that the other did not possess it. Envy operates when another person or group has better gifts, successes, or things, than oneself, making one feel inferior or afraid of the consequences. There is a potentially destructive quality to envy. If I cannot achieve the other's success I will destroy that person's

---

57   See World Health Organization (WHO) (2008) *Closing the Gap in a Generation: Health Equity through Action on the Social Determinants of Health. Final Report of the Commission on Social Determinants of Health.* Geneva: WHO; Department of Health (DoH) (2003) *Tackling Health Inequalities: A Programme for Action.* London: DoH.

58   William Shakespear, *Othello*, act III, scene iii.

59   Garling 2008a, p.416.

60   According to a Finnish study, envy, competition for job status and the inadequate self-image of the perpetrator are suggested as the three main reasons for bullying. Cited by Ministry of Labour (Ireland) (2001) *Report of the Task Force on the Prevention of Workplace Bullying.* Dublin: Government Publications, p.3.

61   George M. Foster (1972) 'The anatomy of envy: A study in symbolic behavior.' *Current Anthropology 13,* 2, 23–29.

62   See Helmut Schoeck (1966) *Envy: A Theory of Social Behaviour.* Indianapolis, IN: Liberty Press, pp.12–16.

reputation through violence such as bullying. Jealousy, on the other hand, is also a potentially destructive sadness. It arises when a person fears losing or has already lost a meaningful status or relationship with another to a rival.[63] Jealousy is often hidden under comments of moral indignation such as 'Who are these people with the impudence to take away what is rightly mine!' The object of jealousy is what the person dreads they might lose, but with envy the spotlight is on the victim, that is, the person is envious of the person lucky enough to possess something held desirable.

These vices thrive in cultures experiencing the unsettling uncertainties of tumultuous change that are characteristic of contemporary healthcare institutions. There is an ongoing struggle for the power to control limited resources. There is the constant risk of losing one's job or being downgraded. Anthropologist George Foster wrote that, in this atmosphere, envy and jealousy thrive because it is thought that someone's gain in terms of prestige and position is possible only because of another's loss.[64] Fed by selfish or narcissistic desires,[65] the envious and the jealous person can become so consumed by anger or rage that nothing else matters but their own world of concern. A climate of suspicion and distrust is created in which deep friendships, collaboration and teamwork become impossible.

Model 6: Blaming culture

Blaming or scapegoating is the process of passionately seeking and marginalizing agents believed to be harming individuals and groups. By transferring the blame for their problems on to others, people are easily able to avoid facing the real causes and the efforts they must make to remove them. Individuals and groups transfer their fears of the unknown and their aggression onto groups or individuals who are visible, relatively powerless, and often already disliked or negatively stereotyped. The greater or more intense the chaos and consequent fear of the unknown, the more likely it is that the powerful emotions of shame, envy, jealousy and fear are operative. For example, one who feels deeply shamed or confused by events, in order to escape an inner sense of inadequacy, may turn in rage on a

---

63   Ibid., pp.115–117.
64   See Foster 1972, pp.165–202.
65   See Neville Symington (1994) *Emotion and Spirit*. London: Cassell, pp.115–127.

person or group that is envied and lay the blame for their problems on innocent others.[66]

Scapegoats hold the pain and suffering for individuals and groups because they can no longer handle it within themselves, but must project and expel it from its midst. The scapegoating process can be swift and merciless; the humanity of the victim must be denied, the victim demonized. The greater or more intense the chaos and consequent fears of the unknown, the more frequent and persistent the scapegoating. The emotions released by the demonizing process makes it difficult for individuals to challenge what is happening; they themselves are liable to become victims also. Only very courageous individuals can stand up to a powerful victim-creating process. Even then, their ability to survive as respected members of the organization is limited.[67]

A *blaming culture* exists whenever scapegoating remains consistently unchallenged by those in authority. A blaming culture destroys trust, fosters an environment of fear and drives people to hide errors lest they be blamed. People become secretive, fearful of trusting others in case they become the targets of blaming. It is assumed that every mistake or error is the result of individual behaviour, rather than the inadequacies of the system. People hesitate to be positive and creative in case their efforts fail; consequently they are marginalized.

CASE STUDY: A BLAMING CULTURE

In 2005 a young Sydney girl died from respiratory arrest due to the depressant effect of opiate medication. It was initially easy to blame the individuals who had administered the wrong drugs, but the coroner found that her death was due to 'poor communication between doctors, staffing inadequacies, no or inadequate medical notes, poor clinical decisions, ignorance of protocols and incorrect decisions by nursing staff'.[68]

---

66 See Stephen Pattison (2000) *Shame: Theory, Therapy, Theology.* Cambridge: Cambridge University Press, pp.116, 127; Arbuckle 2004, pp.136–138.

67 In 2010 Jayant Patel, surgeon, was accused of being responsible for at least 48 serious adverse medical outcomes resulting in at least 13 deaths while employed by the Queensland government. He was eventually convicted of three counts of manslaughter and sentenced to imprisonment. The whistleblower who kept challenging the culture of concealment protecting Patel was marginalized by officials for several years. See Dunbar *et al.* 2011.

68 Garling 2008a, p.6.

Politicians often foster a blaming culture to gain political advantage. In Britain, all parties have felt the need to condemn the quality of the NHS and public services in general to show that if they were in power they would make significant changes. Prime Minister Tony Blair was particularly guilty of using the 'blame language' of the welfare state in order to win support for his reform of the public service, including the NHS. When this happens, hardworking and committed staff are made to feel demeaned, with no way to respond publicly. The present (2011) coalition government's efforts to deregulate the NHS is also playing the blaming game. The thesis of political scientist Francis Fukuyama[69] is that blaming has intensified over the last 30 years simply because 'individualism is less and less curbed by commonly shared values'.[70] Beginning in the 1980s and politically led by President Reagan and Prime Minister Thatcher, the individual moved to centre stage, 'greed became good' and one's obligation to society diminished in importance. For example, Margaret Thatcher tried to wean Britain from the welfare state by privatizing government services, introducing consumers' charters and encouraging the idea of Britons as clients rather than as citizens. This ultimately meant, as sociologist Frank Furedi concluded, that 'individuals have become isolated and vulnerable',[71] and they, not society, are ready targets of blame.

Model 7: Political 'cargo cult' culture

We find millenarian qualities in the style, frequency and radical methods of government 'top-down' bullying interventions in the healthcare systems in England, Australia and New Zealand over the last 30 years. Anthropologically, millenarian movements are noted for their declarations of the end of one age or form of life and the coming or dawning of another more perfect one. In other words, the term 'millennial' describes a wide variety 'of social movements that have in common an aspiration to reform or to overturn the social order with supernatural assistance'.[72] These movements flourish

---

69 See Francis Fukuyama (1995) *Trust: The Social Virtues and the Creation of Prosperity*. London: Hamish Hamilton.

70 Furedi 1997, 8, p.140.

71 Ibid.

72 L. Lindstrom (1996) 'Millennial Movements.' In Alan Barnard and Jonathan Spencer (eds) *Encyclopedia of Social and Cultural Anthropology*. London: Routledge, p.372.

during periods of social, economic and political disruption. Visions of the Nazi new world order or the Marxist classless society are particularly tragic examples of millenarian movements. Less well-known are the past and present 'cargo cult' movements in Melanesia (i.e. Papua New Guinea, Solomon Islands, Vanuatu), in the South Pacific.[73] It is claimed that specified ritual actions and bizarre practices will *suddenly* and *spectacularly* bring their adherents a better, even paradisiacal, life of plenty (called locally 'cargo') under messianic leadership. The 'cargo' message of leaders is: repudiate the past by dramatically destroying crops and other goods as the precondition for the coming of the 'new heaven' of prosperity. When the rituals fail there is great despondency, but new leaders emerge claiming that their predecessors did not have the 'right rituals'; so the cycle of destruction and hollow promises of impressive prosperity begins all over again.

The ways in which healthcare reforms are promoted by politicians often follow a 'cargo cult' pattern. Proposed reforms are presented in a populist style; people are enthusiastically assured that the 'cargo' of better choice and more efficiency, and better services will arrive, provided they vote for the party; previous political leaders are demonized; there is to be the rapid demolition of existing structures. In New Zealand, for example, neoliberal reforms were introduced into the national healthcare system with incredible speed.[74] The business models had been enthusiastically espoused in the late 1980s; politicians promised that if hospitals were conducted as businesses, they would be more efficient and profitable at the same time. Locally elected boards were removed with lightning speed. The promised 'heaven', however, never materialized, so, in the 1990s, local control had to be reintroduced, while the lives of thousands of people had been negatively and needlessly affected by the ideologically led reforms. In England, as this book has already detailed, reform continues to follow reform with breathtaking speed. In the NHS, for example, since the mid-1980s, there has been some significant form of organizational disruption almost annually, due to policy decisions emanating from the Department of Health, with the latest dramatic

---

73 For an example see Peter Lawrence (1964) *Road Belong Cargo: A Study of the Cargo Movement in the Southern Madang District New Guinea.* Manchester: Manchester University Press.
74 See Cheyne *et al.* 2008, pp.222–223, and Gauld 2009.

proposed restructuring in 2010.[75] In New South Wales, Australia, the newly elected Liberal government in 2011 immediately proceeded to demolish examples of the previous government's successful efforts at reform of the public health system, promising to install immediate improvements to the system.

Values-based: Just culture

In contrast to the seven cultural models of bullying, the values-based culture model is designed to prevent intimidating and disruptive behaviours so that people feel trusted and willing to learn from each other and their varied experiences. A just culture model, as applied to healthcare, is a safety-supportive system of shared accountability in which institutions are held responsible for the systems they have created and for encouraging the safe decisions of patients and staff members. In a just culture, errors, hazards, near-misses and critical incidents are reported, so that it is possible to investigate them adequately, learn from them and consequently make improvements. For example, medical error is thought to be the eighth leading cause of death in the United States.[76] In a culture of blame, individuals would be targeted and punished, but the wider failures in the healthcare institutions would be ignored. However, in a just culture, the human errors would be viewed as symptoms of organizational cultural breakdown.[77] The signs of the effectiveness of this model will be:

- The mission is clear and is the primary focus for all decision-making.

- People feel respected and trusted, roles and procedures are clearly defined and accountability systems are fully operative.

- The best method to reduce medical errors is to focus on identifying dysfunctional elements in organizational cultures, rather than primarily blaming the actions of individuals.

---

75 See Department of Health 2010.

76 See Andrew Auerbach, C. Seth Landefeld and Kaveh G. Shojania (2007) 'The tension between needing to improve care and knowing how to do it.' *New England Journal of Medicine* 357, 6, 608.

77 See Sidney Dekker (2007) *Just Culture: Balancing Safety and Accountability.* Farnham: Ashgate, p.131.

○ Leaders expect to receive honest feedback as well as to offer it to those whom they serve; this nurtures trust so people can grow and become creative.

○ Decision-making is based on the principle of subsidiarity, that is, decisions are made, as far as possible, at the point where they are to be implemented. Participative decision-making is the norm, that is, people are appropriately consulted, and listened to, when decisions are to be made.

○ Dialogue is the normal method of resolving conflicts. Dialogue is authentic if three conditions are met: people feel they understand the position of others, they also feel that others understand their points of view, and there is a readiness on the part of all to accept what is decided because it was reached openly and fairly.

○ There is zero tolerance of bullying. People know that their complaints will be immediately taken seriously. Failure to listen to complaints or unnecessary delay in dealing with them is itself an act of bullying.

The ultimate test of the effectiveness of this model is this: do people feel trusted? Trust here is 'a relationship between one or more persons, which has elements of openness and honesty, and a willingness to accept other[s] based on the opinion that the other party is both capable and dependable'.[78] An organizational culture is said to be trusting when there is a kind of collective judgement that the people involved will act with honesty in negotiations, and make 'a good faith effort to behave in accordance with [their] commitments'.[79] Where trust exists, people feel valued, levels of job satisfaction are increased.[80] Trust disintegrates when people fail to be transparently consistent in their behaviour. When I was asked to investigate why the subculture of nurses in one hospital had lost faith in their CEO, I found that, for several years, he had refused to censure a doctor for

78   Rocky J. Dwyer (2008) 'Benchmarking as a process for demonstrating organizational trustworthiness?' *Management Decision 46*, 8, 1211–1212.
79   Ibid.
80   See John Rodwell *et al.* (2009) 'The impact of the work conditions of allied health professionals on satisfaction, commitment and psychological distress.' *Health Care Management Review 34*, 3, 205–293.

his consistent bullying of theatre nurses. Trust was destroyed. The complaining nurses rightly felt that the CEO's failure was a sign of his collusion with the bully. When a new CEO was appointed, the nurses repeated their grievance, not expecting a positive response. In fact, the CEO acted immediately and severely reprimanded the doctor. Trust in the organization was not fully restored until the CEO acted with the same speed over the next two months to remedy other bullying incidents. Trust is something that needs to be earned. That takes time.[81]

Summary

○ Bullies are people with personal inadequacies who project their own fears onto others in order to control them. The impact on their victims, their families and their fellow-workers can be devastating. The Brazilian educationist Paulo Freire writes that: 'In order to dominate, the dominator has no choice but to deny true praxis [i.e. reflective practice] to the people, deny them the right to say their own word and think their own thoughts.'[82] Bullies do not want victims to recount publicly their story of heart-destroying assaults on their dignity, because if they do, they may rediscover what dignity means and, ceasing to be victims, be re-energized to protest against the violence they suffer.

○ Frequently, however, bullies' domination of others is legitimized by the cultures in which they operate. This chapter highlights the types of cultures that legitimize, support or condone bullies. Unless the cultural roots of bullying are firmly addressed it will continue and will remain firmly embedded in cultures. For example, in countries like England, Australia and New Zealand, there is a political culture of bullying in healthcare; it is frequently the target of unnecessary political interference for the primary advantage, not of patients, but of political parties. Employees do not feel valued if they are

---

81   See helpful insights of Susan Groundwater-Smith and Judyth Sachs (2002) 'The activist professional and the reinstatement of trust.' *Cambridge Journal of Education 32*, 3, 67–84.
82   Freire 1972, p.121.

constantly being coerced from above, depending on who is in government and what their agenda happens to be at the moment. Cultures of bullying create stress and reduce staff motivation and discourage creativity. Ultimately, the safety of patients is jeopardized.

○ In contrast to the cultures of bullying, the just culture model is characterized by operative levels of accountability where policies and actions are driven by the mission and values of healthcare; people feel trusted to be creative and to acknowledge their errors in order to improve the safety and welfare of patients. Ultimately, in the just culture people feel their human dignity and that of their colleagues and patients is respected. Of course, since bullying has costly monetary consequences, the more an institution values and promotes a just culture, the more it will benefit financially.

Stratetic implications

Policies

○ Since every person has the right to work in a physically and mentally safe environment, all healthcare institutions must be committed to a policy of 'zero tolerance' for bullying and to the appropriate structures to ensure compliance. However, if foundational values like respect and justice are not being regularly inculcated in in-service training programmes, the policy and structures will be ineffective.

Implementation

○ Complaints need to be rapidly dealt with. Failure to do so sends the message that bullying is not being taken seriously. All staff members must be required to attend professionally led anti-bullying workshops.

○ There must be supportive structures to ensure the job security and the general well-being of whistleblowers, that is, those who report incidents of bullying.

○ Each staff member has the obligation to critique the way they behave and speak to others because they can even unintentionally be acting in a bullying manner. This is especially important, as healthcare institutions are increasingly being staffed by members of different ethnic groups.

○ Derogatory or bullying language can involve not just jokes about other ethnic or minority groups, but also the use of emotion-charged, deeply offensive stereotypical words to describe different ethnic groups. The object of an ethnic joke is to 'put down' members of a certain group while, at the same time, implicitly presenting one's own group as superior. Such jokes, while appearing to be funny, reinforce the culture of bullying. The same warning applies to sexist language. Male-centred cultures also contain words that assume and reinforce an inferior status for women and they can be used without people realizing their offensive and unjust connotations.[83] Individuals and groups that are sensitive to this abusive language have the power to stop its use.[84]

○ Managers need to pay particular attention to incidents of bullying of junior clinicians by their seniors; this will involve a process of empowering junior doctors to feel safe in reporting such episodes.

○ Individuals who are the targets of bullying should be aware of their legal rights, avoid confronting the bully alone, if possible, and seek advice and help from trustworthy people, who are in a position of at least equal seniority to the bully. Since counsellors who are employed by an organization must ultimately be loyal to it, it is often wiser for victims to seek professional help outside the organization.

---

83 Geri-Ann Galanti warns that 'male physicians from male-dominated countries tend to be even more domineering than American male doctors, and female nurses from such countries tend to be more submissive than American nurses': (1997) *Caring for Patients from Different Cultures: Case Studies from American Hospitals,* 2nd edn. Philadelphia, PA: University of Pennsylvania Press, p.92.

84 A small group of people in New Zealand once complained to the Race Relations Office about a national competition for the best Irish jokes initiated by a supposedly reputable weekly newspaper. The paper immediately ceased to publish the jokes.

○ There are steps that non-victims can take to assist victims of bullying:

- Listen attentively to the victim's story. Gently encourage them to describe what has happened, reassuring them that they are safe with you.

- Speak up when people are being bullied; whistleblowing is always risky so people need to seek advice and support before they act.

- Since a bully can artfully undermine or destroy the self-confidence of a victim, be sure to encourage the victim's self-worth, not in a general way, but by pointing out specific examples of the person's competence.

CHAPTER 5

Leading Cultural Change in Healthcare

Culture is created... embedded and strengthened by leaders.
(Edgar H. Schein)[1]

This chapter explains:

○ that management is commonly confused with leadership

○ that cultural change in healthcare requires a particular type of leaders, namely *paramodern leaders*

○ that paramodern leaders committed to cultural change in healthcare institutions possess particular qualities such as: imagination, creativity, collaborative skills and a willingness to return to the founding story of healthcare and its values.

The purpose of this chapter is to clarify the meaning of leadership and then to describe the particular type of *paramodern* leadership that is required to lead cultural change in healthcare based on its residual founding story and values (see Chapter 2). Leaders need to be sensitive to the dynamics of culture and the role of storytelling as the driving force of cultural change. As Edgar Schein observes, 'leadership and culture management are so central to understanding organizations and making them effective that we cannot afford to be complacent about either one'.[2]

Professional reports on the future of healthcare institutions broadly indicate that leadership and cultural change are necessary for their transformation. Thomas H. Lee, a professor of medicine at Harvard Medical School, is correct when he writes that 'Taming [the] chaos [of healthcare] requires a new breed of leaders at every level.'[3]

---

1   Schein 1985, pp.316–317.
2   Ibid., p.327.
3   Lee 2010, p.53.

In particular, however, leadership in healthcare 'must come substantially from doctors and other clinicians, whether or not they play formal management roles'.[4] What is meant by leadership in the literature is, however, often confused with management.[5] For example, in 2000 the Department of Health in London, in setting out the plan for the future of the NHS, claimed that: 'We need clinical and managerial leaders through the health service',[6] yet the document fails to define this precisely. Often the problem of leadership is seen to be a political and monetary issue: if more money could be put into the system all would be well. Yet no matter how much money is made available, the primary and urgent challenge confronting people in any healthcare institution remains the same: to find ways of working collaboratively together and resolving 'the problems out on the ground'.[7]

The second point of agreement is that healthcare systems must undergo cultural change if they are to respond to changing needs. Thus, 'extending employee engagement is not an issue for legislation or regulation: it requires cultural change. More people need to "get it" – and more people need to do it.'[8] All staff members must become champions of cultural change.[9] One NHS document stated: 'We want to create a culture in the NHS which celebrates and encourages success and innovation.'[10] An excellent aspiration but, as explained in Chapter 1, sustained cultural change is fraught with many complex difficulties, especially in massive and highly complex organizations like contemporary healthcare systems.

CASE STUDY: LEADERSHIP CHALLENGE

Figures 5.1 and 5.2 illustrate the extent of the challenge confronting not just the public health system of New South Wales, Australia, as shown, but every contemporary healthcare system: how to promote and maintain

---

4   Mountford and Webb 2009, 9; see also Garling 2008b, pp.11–12.
5   See for example Department of Health (2000b) *The NHS Plan: A Plan for Investment, A Plan for Reform.* London: Stationery Office, pp.86–87; Parkin 2009, pp.88–89.
6   Department of Health 2000b, p.87.
7   See Gerry Robinson (2007) *The Challenges of Leadership in the NHS.* London: NHS Confederation, p.2.
8   David MacLeod and Nita Clarke (2009) *Engaging for Success: Enhancing Performance through Employee Engagement.* Kew: Office of Public Sector Information, p.117.
9   See Garling 2008b, p.4.
10   Department of Health (DoH) (1998) *A First Class Service: Quality in the New NHS.* London: DoH, p.72. See excellent discussion of this issue by Parkin 2009, pp.115–117.

the founding mission and values of healthcare as the driving force in decision-making and action (see Chapter 2), while being constrained at the same time within budget limits. CEOs and other executives face increasingly enormous leadership challenges. Figure 5.1 provides an overview of the culture as described by Commissioner Peter Garling, in an exhaustive probing report into the public healthcare system in New South Wales in 2008. The values listed under 'the mission' are either explicitly or implicitly those of the founding story of healthcare; the report indicated a definite myth drift away from the original values of healthcare namely: compassion, respect, equity, justice, collaboration and dialogue. The primary emphasis, as the report noted, is more on 'the business' pole of the tension, with its undue concern for meeting targets, micro-management from the top,[11] clinical self-interested silos,[12] the dramatic split between managers and clinicians, a system noted for bullying at all levels, lack of trust, compassion and respect, and unwillingness to celebrate success of individuals and groups.[13] The report forcefully concluded that the health system had become so dysfunctional that, 'a new culture needs to take root which sees the patient's needs as the paramount central concern of the system',[14] or the entire state-wide system may not survive.[15]

Split		
The Mission............................		....................**The Business**
Weak stress on values		**Strong stress on values**
Compassion		Targets
Respect		Top-down
Solidarity		Biomedical
Justice		Individualism
Equity		
Dialogue		**Results**
Collaboration		Chaos
		Siloisms
		Splitting
		Bullying

Figure 5.1: Model 1: NSW Health: biomedical/corporate culture

11 See Garling 2008b, pp.31–32.
12 Ibid., p.4.
13 Ibid., p.11.
14 Ibid., p.3.
15 Ibid.

The New South Wales State government swiftly reacted by publishing *Caring Together*, an action plan approving 134 of the 139 recommendations of the original report and establishing an independent panel to ensure their implementation.[16] Figure 5.2 summarizes what the changed nature of the healthcare culture should look like if the reforms are effectively implemented. The government's plan is to return the primary emphasis in the cultures of the acute care hospitals to their founding stories and values through leaders, or champions, at all levels of the system. Thus, in anthropological terms, the government is hoping for a mythological revitalization process to take place; economic rationalism is to give way to fundamental human values of compassion, respect, solidarity, equity, justice, collaboration and dialogue. Making the cultural shift from Model 1 to Model 2 successfully will take several years of risky and challenging work, demanding appropriate leadership and management at all levels.

The Mission driving..The Business	
Strong stress on values	**Strong emphasis on**
Patient-centred care	Clinician-driven leadership
Respect	Subsidiarity
Compassion	Teamwork
Equity	Accountability
Social	Innovation
Collaboration	Anti-bullying
Dialogue	Anti-soloism

Figure 5.2: Model 2: NSW Government reform proposal

Leadership: Terminology and styles

Terminology: Variety

Bookshelves are today groaning under the weight of more and more publications on the nature and art of leadership. These books come with an array of bewildering terms and catchphrases, for

---

16   See NSW Government (2009) *Caring Together: The Health Action Plan for NSW.* Sydney: NSW Department of Health.

example: 'situational leadership', 'hands-on, value-driven',[17] 'heroes of innovation', 'rites and rituals of leaders in corporate cultures',[18] 'champions of change', 'intrapreneurs',[19] 'transformative and transactional leaders'[20] and, more recently, 'humble leadership' and 'bottom-up leadership'.[21] According to 'situational leadership' the success of a leader depends on the willingness of a group to choose leaders able to take on the style of leading most suited to the overall purpose of the group at a particular time. That is, there are occasions in which the leader needs to delegate, persuade, provide directives or foster participation/collaboration.[22] Where what has to be done is uncertain or ill focused, as will be the case in times of change, such as in contemporary healthcare, in which considerable innovative skills are required, a transforming style of leadership is necessary – one based on trust and mutuality. The task of the transforming leader is primarily to foster a collaborative or participative atmosphere in which this trust and mutuality exist as prerequisites for creative action or strategies for change.[23]

Peter Block uses the words 'governance' and 'stewardship' instead of 'leadership' in order to avoid any connotations of the patriarchal, control model of management. For him, governance is the way we define the purpose of our organization. It defines also *how* we are to use its power and resources.[24] 'Stewardship' is at the heart of governance. By stewardship Block means 'accountability without control or compliance'.[25] It means that there can be no authentic reform of an organization unless people are prepared to make an appropriate change of values from self-interest to concern for the welfare of others. He correctly insists that it is insufficient just to change structures and expect that reform will follow; rather the fundamental

17 See Tom J. Peters and Robert H. Waterman (1982) *In Search of Excellence: Lessons from America's Best-Run Companies.* New York: Harper & Row.

18 See Terrence E. Deal and Allan A. Kennedy (1982) *Corporate Cultures: The Rites and Rituals of Corporate Life.* Reading, MA: Addison-Wesley.

19 See Gifford Pinchot (1985) *Intrapreneuring.* New York: Harper & Row.

20 See James M. Burns (1978) *Leadership.* New York: Harper Torch, pp.149–192.

21 See 'The shackled boss' (2012) *The Economist* (21 January), 68.

22 See Paul Hersey and Ken Blanchard (1982) *Management of Organizational Behavior: Utilizing Human Resources.* Englewood Cliffs, NJ: Prentice Hall.

23 See John Heap (1989) *The Management of Innovation and Design.* London: Cassell, pp.69–75.

24 See Peter Block (1993) *Stewardship: Choosing Service over Self-Interest.* San Francisco, CA: Berrett-Koehler, p.5.

25 Ibid., p.xx.

belief system of an organization must change – from self-interest and individualism to solidarity and collaboration.[26] This is what others term 'servant-leadership'[27] to emphasize the importance of openness and persuasion, not control or coercion. Servant leadership is not about a personal search for power, prestige or material rewards. Instead, servant leadership starts with the motivation to serve others. Rather than controlling or wielding power, the servant leader aims to build a firm foundation or shared goals by listening deeply to understand the needs and concerns of others, working attentively to help build consensus. In recent times the terms 'social innovative leaders'[28] and 'social entrepreneurial leaders'[29] have become popular, particularly when referring to partnerships of the for-profits and the non-profit sectors. Social innovators are skilled leaders who are able to develop fresh strategies, concepts and ideas. They lead organizations that respond to social needs of all kinds, such as healthcare, and that extend and reinforce civil society. Despite the diversity of language, the following theoretical threads about the reform of organizations run through these terms:

○ Change is a fact of life and leadership for change must be an integral part of all organizations if they are to survive and grow.

○ Today, the emphasis in leadership has moved from management in order to control groups to a transforming or refounding style that aims to bring the best out of people and to respond quickly to rapid change.

○ A leader moulds and communicates a task-oriented mission and vision which gives direction to the work of others; if the leader fails to provide the mission and vision, the strategies to realize it and appropriate accountability structures, the group becomes confused and de-energized.

---

26   Ibid., p.103.
27   See Robert K. Greenleaf (1977) *Servant Leadership: A Journey into the Nature of Legitimate Power and Greatness.* New York: Paulist.
28   See Stephen Goldsmith (2010) *The Power of Social Innovation.* San Francisco, CA: Jossey-Bass.
29   See Charles Leadbeater (1997) *The Rise of the Social Entrepreneur.* London: Demos, and Andrew Mawson (2008) *The Social Entrepreneur.* London: Atlantic Books.

○ Leaders, in shaping the mission and vision of an organization, must involve members of the organization in a collaborative way. Leaders must have the ability themselves and with the help of others to strategize their vision into concrete plans for action.

○ Leaders must realize that people belong to cultures that tend more to obstruct creativity and change (see Chapter 1).

○ Leaders, who seek cultural change, cannot succeed unless they themselves and their followers are prepared to change their values and attitudes; that is, structural change alone will not lead to cultural change.

○ Leaders empower others to act, by encouraging collaboration and by building an atmosphere of trust and respect for human dignity; they recognize the gifts of others and celebrate their achievements.[30]

○ Leaders call people to be accountable for their behaviour according to the mission, vision and strategies they have accepted.

In order to appreciate, however, the difficulties in defining leadership it is important to identify the historical philosophical influences that affect the way leaders actually operate.

Leadership styles: Background

The three philosophical and sociological movements in the Western world that particularly influence the way people define leadership are modernity, postmodernity and paramodernity.

Modernity

Since the sixteenth century the leader's role and the traditional style of management in healthcare organizations has been significantly influenced by the assumptions of classical physicist Isaac Newton (see Chapter 2) and the philosopher John Locke (1632–1704). Newton depicted a clockwork universe governed by unchanging

---

30   See James M. Kouzes and Barry Z. Posner (1990) *The Leadership Challenge*. San Francisco, CA: Jossey-Bass, pp.279–280.

laws, while Locke believed there were laws of nature controlling human society similar to the laws described by Newton. Terms that best describe the Lockean ideal society are stability, equilibrium, predictability and order. Feelings have no place in maintaining order as they distract from the real work of rational thinking and planning. The aim of leadership is to obtain rational agreement to logically presented decisions. People who dare to rebel against rationally presented arguments and decisions must be marginalized because they endanger order. Patriarchy and Social Darwinism have been additional powerful forces in shaping modernity. It was assumed that only men could undertake logical, rational or emotionless thinking. Qualities viewed as feminine, such as intuition, nurturing and empathic support, were signs of weakness. Social Darwinism holds that individuals and societies were destined by nature to compete for survival; only the strong would continue and the weak would die out. Weak individuals and societies must not be helped to survive because this would hold back the strong from their rightful progress. Organizations must be hierarchical in order to allow the most skilled (mainly men or women who think like men!) to rule from the top and to control the weak beneath them. Thus, according to modernity thinking, the primary task of healthcare leaders is to make decisions that foster and maintain orderly relationships in their institutions.[31] They bask in their clarity of thinking because, to them, whatever is confused, disorderly or chaotic is 'unnatural' and is to be considered dangerous to the survival of an organization.

Postmodernity

The terms 'postmodernity' and 'postmodernism' are freely used today, but without being defined in any consistent way; both terms have become elastic and, for many, disturbingly elusive.[32] In this book, however, postmodernity refers to a way of thinking and acting that has cast aside most of the cultural certainties and optimism of modernity. Emerging as a cultural force in the 1950s and 1960s, postmodernity rejects the assumptions that reality is so structured

31   See Reuben R. McDaniel (1997) 'Strategic leadership: A view from quantum and chaos theories.' *Health Care Management Review 22*, 1, 21–37.
32   See Anthony Giddens (1990) *The Consequences of Modernity*. Cambridge: Polity Press; Ernest Gellner (1992) *Postmodernism, Reason and Religion*. London: Routledge, p.22; Arbuckle 2004, pp.154–162.

that it can be uncovered by the human mind through rational and logical methods, and that it is possible to build a universal culture upon the foundation of rational thought. While the mythology of postmodernity has many positive qualities, for example, the ability to critique the trappings of patriarchy and social elitism, it is also characterized by negative features, such as an extensive malaise notable for its cynicism, pragmatism, narcissism and scepticism. In summary, the particularly significant elements of postmodernity are lack of depth and fragmentation. Depth has been replaced by multiple surfaces. There are no hidden meanings; indeed, there is nothing beneath the glittering surfaces that this culture presents. History is meaningless, just a method to give false security or identity to people and a way to obtain power over others. Human relations are fragmentary. There is no longer any meaningful basis for collective agreement or collective action, as the only thing that exists is the self, although the true self is unknowable.

Postmodernity is not a foundation on which to build a community in which people are concerned about others; individuals join an organization primarily for their own ends, and any commitment to serve the common good is considered a waste of time. It is then useless for leaders, for example, in healthcare, to appeal to history or universal values like compassion, equity or justice because they simply cannot exist. No rules are tolerated that in any way bind the individual to a sense of order. It is futile to draw people's attention to the unconscious influence of myths because they are considered to be mere figments of the imagination. Only what one sees on the surface is real, and even that is doubtful.

Paramodernity

The term 'paramodernity' connotes contemporary ways of thinking and acting in reaction to the excessive optimism and rationality of modernity on the one hand, and, on the other, the built-in pessimism and self-destructiveness of much postmodernist thinking. Paramodernity, where 'we glimpse new ways of thinking about ourselves, new possibilities for coexisting with others – even profoundly different others',[33] is very slowly and hesitantly emerging

---

33   Walter T. Anderson (1995) *The Truth about Truth: De-confusing and Re-constructing the Postmodern World.* New York: Putnam, p.11.

as an influential culture model. Values such as holistic health, care for the environment, dialogue, collaboration, compassion and justice are seen to be critically important. Paramodernists assume that the movement of change is not smooth, but lurching, and the necessary impetus or catalyst is stress or cultural chaos, that is, the radical breakdown of predictability. Instead of a machine-like universe of modernity, the world is understood in terms of relationships between living organisms that are essentially cooperative and characterized by coexistence, relational interdependence and symbiosis. Touch one relationship within an organizational culture and all are affected to some degree. Leaders, therefore, need to think in terms of cultural systems. All aspects of an organizational culture, such as we find in healthcare systems, are interrelated or connected in a thoroughly complex network.[34] Contrary to Newtonian thought, most relationships are non-linear, that is, irregular, capricious, messy, unpredictable, chaotic.[35] Systems are inherently unstable,[36] but these systemic instabilities are not random, because there is a pattern within them based on orderly principles which are termed 'strange attractors'.

CASE STUDY: MEDICAL APPLICATION

While physics is not able to foresee what will happen in nature, it nonetheless can provide ways to influence the way we live. One technical function of the chaos theory in medicine is a better understanding of heart fibrillation. When the heart begins to flutter as a result of a mechanism that is explicable in chaos terms, a defibrillator gives it a good push with an electric shock to disrupt the chaotic process and set it right again.[37]

---

34 See McDaniel 1997, 25; Addie Fuhriman and Gary M. Burlingame (1994) 'Measuring small group process: A methodological application of chaos theory.' *Small Group Research 25*, 4, 504.

35 See Bernice Cohen (1997) *The Edge of Chaos: Financial Booms, Bubbles, Crashes and Chaos.* Chichester: Wiley, p.81. The defibrillator works by stopping all intrinsic electrical activity, causing asystole (that is, cardiac arrest). The heart has no electrical activity until the pacemakers start again. This is analogous to jumping up in the middle of a meeting and shouting 'Stop' or a strike walk out. If the pacemakers are abnormal and not synchronized, a person gets fibrillation again.

36 See 'Balancing broomsticks.' (1994) *The Economist* (25 June), 85.

37 See Mark Buchanan (1998) 'Fascinating rhythm.' *New Scientist 157*, 215, 20–25.

According to this culture model strategic leaders in healthcare today must therefore abandon any fixation with undue control and stability and the assumption that one person alone can achieve meaning in chaos. This means fostering as wide a participation in decision-making as is possible.[38] Chaos brings an opportunity to innovate. Yet, to make use of chaos, there must be diversity of thinking. This means cultivating conversations between people of different professional backgrounds within the organization, for example, conversations in healthcare between managers and clinicians, between clinicians and clinicians. Decisions are not to be made without ample opportunity for brainstorming; this allows people time and space to use their intuitive intelligence to gain insights into reality, creativity and change. When leadership is collaborative, trust develops, people feel respected and willingly commit themselves to find solutions in chaotic situations. Once trust exists, an organization is able to devote most of its energies productively, instead of to its own internal battles for power.

Integral to paramodernity is the desire for storytelling as a means to achieve personal and community identities (see Chapter 1). In describing this process of storytelling or narrating, Anthony Giddens commented that 'the narrative of self has in fact to be continually re-worked, and lifestyle practices brought into line with it'.[39] As individuals construct stories from experience, so also will groups of all kinds: business organizations, communities, governments and nations assemble preferred narratives that tell them who they are at this moment in time, where they come from, what is good or bad, and how to organize themselves and maintain their sense of unique identity in a changing world.

---

38 See Margaret J. Wheatley (1992) *Leadership and the New Science: Learning about Organization from an Orderly Universe*. San Francisco, CA: Berret-Koehler, p.64; Ralph D. Stacey (1993) *The Chaos Frontier: Creative Strategic Control for Business*. Oxford: Butterworth-Heinemann, pp.153–230; Michael L. Heifetz (1993) *Leading Change, Overcoming Chaos*. Berkeley, CA: Ten Speed Press, pp.99–132; Susan M. Campbell (1995) *From Chaos to Confidence*. New York: Simon & Schuster, pp.197–225.

39 Anthony Giddens (1992) *The Transformation of Intimacy: Sexuality, Love and Eroticism in Modern Societies*. Cambridge: Polity Press, p.75.

Paramodern leadership in healthcare

The focus of the remainder of this chapter is on the role of the paramodern leader in healthcare. In a chaotically changing world, the paramodern leader in healthcare is able to inspire people in a collaborative way:

○ to create a new imaginative vision of reality, based on the mission and values of the original founding story of healthcare

○ and to work together to bring this vision into reality through concrete strategies

○ thus enabling people to foster within themselves their own creative potential for ongoing cultural change for the benefit of people.

This definition of paramodern leaders and their qualities will now be explained under a series of headings and with particular reference to the following very simple case study of paramodern leadership. Readers surely could recount experiences like the one depicted. Paramodern leaders in healthcare have distinctive qualities, for example, inspired by its founding story they are collaborative, committed to accountability, financially competent, imaginatively proactive, courageous, appreciative of the different gifts of their colleagues and committed to the importance of storytelling as a way of binding people together in a common mission.[40]

CASE STUDY: PARAMODERN LEADERSHIP

One of the earliest memories of my mother in New Zealand during the war was riding a bicycle along rough country roads in total darkness, sometimes even in heavy rain. The village where we lived was seven miles from a hospital in the nearest town, but because of the shortage of doctors and limited transport facilities people in the village were deprived of medical assistance. My mother as a trained nurse decided on her own initiative to do something about it. She, having vainly tried to interest the hospital authorities in the plight of the villagers, started to visit and nurse needy sick people, using her bicycle as the only means

40   See Arbuckle 2000, pp.209–210.

of transport then available and offering whatever help she could. She asked nothing in return. Often she was called out during the blackout hours and off she would go, ignoring the physical dangers of riding in total darkness. Over time she developed a small group of local people as supporters. I remember listening to a family friend asking my mother why she did this. Her reply was quite simple: 'I do this because this is what the Good Samaritan with his compassion and concern for others would have done and moreover this is what Michael Savage was on about when he as prime minister established our welfare system!' My mother continued to pester the medical authorities at the hospital for more help, even if this meant riding her bicycle on the lonely road to the hospital to plead her case. She gently but firmly kept reminding officials that public hospitals must exemplify the qualities of the Good Samaritan inherent in the founding story of the New Zealand welfare system: compassion, solidarity, concern for the marginalized. Eventually they assisted her with medicines and in other ways.

Authority, power and leadership

Leadership is here defined as the process of influencing the action of an individual or a group in an effort to achieve a goal in a given situation. 'Leadership' is an *effort* to influence, but 'power' is a leader's *potential* to influence; 'authority' is the legitimacy to exercise power. Of the many types of authority, 'position authority' is the most commonly discussed. This is the authority to use the power flowing from a person's status within an organization, such as the power that accompanies the office of the administrators of the hospital in the above example. The second type is termed 'personal authority'. This is legitimacy to influence others because of one's personal gifts. My mother possessed personal power, but at the same time she had authority to challenge the hospital's officials, not from any formally recognized position, but from her commitment to the mission of the government hospital. Using her personal power my mother balanced four functions, namely, the functions of conserving, managing, nurturing or empowering others, and pro-acting. She exercised a conserving function by passionately identifying with the heart of the founding experience of healthcare, in her case, the Good Samaritan story and its inherent values. She managed by using her collaborative and conversational style in the manner in which she encouraged others to help. And the latter were empowered to use their skills to support the project. Finally, she was proactive. She created the opportunity to bridge the gap between the founding myth and the contemporary reality of the hospital's initial lack of concern for rural people.

Mission, values, vision

Paramodern leaders are able to articulate and communicate to an organization its mission, values, vision and strategies in a collaborative way. At the same time, they call people to be accountable for their actions. Leaders will ensure that the mission and vision statements of an organization are realistic and adhered to. An organization's *mission statement*, which will contain the values of the organization, will distinguish the organization from all others of its type by asking and collaboratively answering the questions: 'Who are we?' and 'What do we do?' The mission statement will be sufficiently inspirational to empower people to act when leaders, with position or personal authority, passionately believe in it. Such was the case with my mother; she ardently believed that the hospital should be living out the mission and values of the Good Samaritan story.

Since the only constant in today's economic, political and social world is change and the 'only stability possible is stability in motion',[41] paramodern leaders in healthcare will recognize that an organization's founding mission and values are the critical 'strange attractors'. They provide the necessary stability in the midst of change. No organization, including healthcare, can ignore the reality of radical uncertainty at the heart of all change. Charles Handy, the management writer, believes that 'chaotic and energetic but uncontrolled organizations [as in healthcare] can exhibit movement without meaning unless they have found their strange attractor, which gives them point and purpose'. The strange attractor is the '"soul" of the organization.' The 'principal task of leadership', he continues, '[is] to find the strange attractor which will give meaning'[42]

41   John W. Gardner, cited by Robert H. Waterman (1987) *The Renewal Factor*. New York: Bantam, p.213.
42   Charles Handy (1977) 'Unimagined Futures.' In Marshall Goldsmith, Frances Hesselbein and Richard Beckhard (eds) *The Leader of the Future*. San Francisco, CA: Jossey-Bass, p.381.

in the midst of the chaos. The 'strange attractors' in the midst of the turmoil that confronts healthcare organizations are the mission and the values inherent in the residual founding mythology of healthcare in the Western world, namely that of the Good Samaritan. The task of leadership is to rearticulate these values inherent in the story in such a way that people are uplifted and moved to apply its lessons to the contemporary world of healthcare. Unless there are leaders who, operating out of these values, are able to inspire professionals to abandon their defensive cultural barriers, then high-quality, cost-effective patient care based on the values of respect and solidarity will never be achieved and sustained.[43]

Vision is defined as a mental passage from the known to the unknown, creating the future from a mass of existing facts, hopes, dreams, dangers and opportunities. A vision statement articulates a mutual purpose or everyone's agreed destination in response to the question: 'What do we want this team to look like within a set period of time?' A realistic vision statement must be sharply focused. Otherwise, strategic planning to realize the vision will be fuzzy. If there is no clear vision, the group becomes confused and de-energized. A *strategy* is a plan for the use of resources in order to implement in concrete terms a group's vision. My mother had a clear vision of how people in rural areas needing healthcare should be treated. She then deliberately strategized by getting to know people at the hospital and winning over a group of local supporters, and deciding to act at the appropriate times.

Leadership and management: Differing roles

In England, when the authors of the NHS documents refer to leadership, they in fact really mean management. This is, unfortunately, a common confusion.[44] The primary task of a manager is to prevent the complexity of a modern organizational culture degenerating into total chaos. Managers are responsible for areas of financial planning, quality control, staffing and market research, and give order and consistency to them. For managers, the smooth running of systems and structures are the essentials, and change is not integral to their

---

43   See Shortell *et al.* 2000, p.85.
44   See Allsop 1995, pp.42–59.

role. The manager bows to the status quo, but the paramodern leader challenges the status quo to face up to change in the environment. A manager's role is to maintain order, formulate strategic goals and allocate resources according to the vision. As leadership adviser Warren Bennis commented: 'The manager maintains; the leader develops...The manager relies on control; the leader inspires trust... The manager has his [sic] eye on the bottom line; the leader has his eye on the horizon.'[45] Understood in this way, we need both leadership *and* management. Again, Stephen Covey wrote: 'Management is doing things right; leadership is doing the right things. Management is efficiency in climbing the ladder of success; leadership determines which ladder is leaning against the right wall.'[46] In my mother's example, the hospital officials needed to be gently but persistently challenged to re-own their position authority (which they did).

Collaborative leadership for cultural change

The driver in cultural change is collaborative leadership that focuses on mission, vision and strategies. If people do not see the need for change, then even the use of coercive power has limited impact in the long term. Time spent involving people in the change process both respects their dignity and is a precondition to effective cultural change. My mother was aware of this, so she spent significant time winning the support of people around her and then of the hospital officials. No one person can be absolutely certain that their mission, vision and strategies are appropriate; they need collaborative action for thinking them through. As Paul Parkin, a writer on change management, commented, in healthcare today, the '"great man" theory of the single charismatic leader, developed from Nietzsche's conception of 'superman'so beloved by politicians and the head-hunter industry is outdated and a mistake'.[47]

Collaborative leadership is the result of a high level of *interdependency*, that is, the paramodern leader will ensure that each person in the team has their role clarified and feels responsible for, and is supported in, its achievement, but works to combine their

45   Warren Bennis (1989) *On Becoming a Leader*. Reading, MA: Addison-Wesley, p.45.
46   Stephen Covey (1990) *The Seven Habits of Highly Effective People: Powerful Lessons in Personal Change*. New York: Simon & Schuster, p.101.
47   Parkin 2009, p.94.

actions with those of others in view of a commonly accepted vision and mission. In my experience of healthcare systems, the failure to clarify roles is a source of unnecessary turmoil and frustration. The collaborative approach also means that all team members share in the decision-making process. They may do this in one of several ways, for example, discussion leads to consensus or a majority vote or the team leader decides after consultation with other members. The preference is for the first option: full involvement in decision-making through consensus. However, there must be flexibility. The group should learn what option is the most appropriate at a given time. For example, urgency for a decision and action may only allow that a decision is made by the one with the most authority. If lengthy and wide consultation or majority voting is mandatory, then decisions may never be made and urgent needs are left unattended. True consensus occurs after all parties feel they have been involved at each stage and that their views have been considered. There may be disagreement over the details of the decision, but all accept that it is the best in the circumstances.

However, if consensus decision-making is pursued at all costs – that is, if it is made into a rigid ideology – then points of conflict and disagreement can be forced underground. If attention is not paid to these issues then all kinds of unresolved negative feelings or hurts will haunt the group and threaten to split it apart at some point later. Sometimes, there is unnecessary tension when team members are not informed of the type of participation before their advice is sought: is it simple consultation, consensus or majority vote? False expectations can be raised, and then distrust – the enemy of collaboration – emerges. Pseudo-consultation, involving the illusion of participation without the substance, is to be avoided. Leaders have already made decisions, but other team members are then 'consulted to keep them happy'. There is no intention of changing the original decisions. From my experience of healthcare institutions, pseudo-consultation can be all too frequent. It leads to the breakdown of trust of those in authority, disillusionment, disaffection, cynicism and comments like: 'I know their mind was already made up before I was even asked. What's the use of trying!'

Diversity of gifts

The team to lead culture change needs to possess a variety of qualities, as helpfully explained by Ned Herrmann, researcher into creative thinking. He described these qualities by clarifying four different ways people think and act: 'machine-gun thinkers', 'detail thinkers', 'storytellers' and 'dreamers'.[48] While an individual may use all four patterns, he or she may prefer one mode of thinking in a specific situation. While my mother had all four qualities she particularly exemplified gifts of storytelling and dreaming. 'Machine-gun thinkers' are highly rational and quick thinkers – analytical, factual and precise – and stress the major points of issues. People like lawyers, physicians, financial officers and scientists tend to be machine-gun thinkers. 'Detail thinkers' are present-oriented people, logical and slow thinkers, concerned with detailed information, but poor at seeing patterns in such material. They make effective accountants, middle-managers, quality control agents, site managers. A machine-gun thinker will tell people the nature of the end product, but the detail thinker explains step-by-step how the product is to be realized.

'Storytellers' are intuitive, deeply concerned with the feelings of people, stressing teamwork, relationships and participation in group activities. They are the recounters of anecdotes that remind people of founding stories and the heroes of organizations. Social workers, nurses, teachers and personnel officers tend to be storytellers.

CASE STUDY: HOSPITAL STORYTELLERS

As a patient in hospitals, I quickly discovered who were the very effective storytellers. I recall, for example, several people, who while regularly cleaning my room or preparing for my meals, would take time to chat with me, asking how I was progressing, cheerfully recounting stories of patients they had known with the same problems as myself and how they had recovered, and why they liked working at the hospital. I recall also the compassionate ways in which people admitted me to the hospitals, together with the nurses who directly cared for me. Unselfconsciously, these people were both articulating and living the

---

48   See summary of Ned Herrmann's analysis in Neuhauser 1988, pp.71–85.

values of the hospital's mission. When hospitals fail to attract people with these gifts, they become mere technical machines. They lose the foundational story for their existence.

'Dreamers' are well attuned to work with chaos, as their thinking is not linear. They are more intuitive than logical and factual. They are future-oriented, highly imaginative people, with new ideas springing from a mind that organizes experiences, facts and relationships to discern a path that has not been taken before. Somewhere along this uncharted path, intuition compresses years of learning and experience into an instantaneous flash.[49] They are rarely able to provide, before a project begins, all the concrete details for its implementation. They act in short stages, then evaluate and change direction with ease if it appears that is the right thing to do. As their thinking does not follow predictable patterns, they can feel oppressed by routine or the acceptable order of 'doing things around here'. Artists, architects, entrepreneurs and strategic thinkers are 'dreamers who act', that is, they have the added gift of being able to strategize their vision through concrete action. Herrmann highlighted the tensions that can exist between people who use different thinking and acting modes. For example, dreamers and storytellers cause considerable anxiety and annoyance to machine-gun and detail thinkers – and vice versa. Little wonder that medical clinicians find storytelling team members annoying! Yet each mode is essential for good teamwork if change is to be sensitively led.

Empowering

Paramodern leaders empower people to become more active, more creative in the control of their lives and institutions through interacting with others in trust and mutuality. They set direction in a collaborative way, as my mother did in her unassuming way, fostering discussions of values, enfranchising people in decision-making, building coalitions that achieve goals in a proactive way, inspiring and motivating others.[50] Psychologist Gordon Lawrence distinguished between leaders acting by the 'politics of salvation' and

49   See Roy Rowan (1986) *The Intuitive Manager*. New York: Berkley, pp.11–14.
50   See Duncan *et al*. 1995, p.465.

those by the 'politics of revelation'. Leaders of the first type exercise their leadership in order to 'rescue' or 'save' people from oppressive structures without really consulting or drawing on the experience and expertise of the people themselves. Sometimes leadership of this type is necessary, but the danger is that it can become the normal way of acting instead of the exception. Paramodern leaders, however, prefer to act according to the criteria of the 'politics of revelation', that is, they aim to develop those processes that encourage the responsible exercise of authority, both individually and collectively, so that people become generative of ideas and the agents of their own growth and that of the group.[51]

CASE STUDY: INTEGRATIVE VERSUS NUTRITIVE AUTHORITY

In the mid-1960s I researched the reasons for the successful development of credit unions (small-scale people's banks) in Fiji, in the South Pacific, under the direction of Marion Ganey. Their prosperity contrasted with the frequent failures of the cooperative movement initiated and directed by a paternalistic colonial government. The behaviour of the government's cooperative officials exemplified 'structures of salvation'. They acted *for* the people, refusing to believe that the Fijian people could ever run their own affairs. On the other hand, Ganey's success in establishing credit unions was due to two factors: his ability to impart, in a trusting way, a vision of a people able to run their own lives, and the establishment of 'structures of revelation' through which people could claim their own authority to decide for themselves how they are to live. One informant summarized Ganey's leadership skills: 'When he comes into the village we all feel ten feet taller and ten years younger! When government agents come, however, we are made to feel like children!'

This case study can be further enlightened by a distinction made by Rollo May. He distinguishes between 'nutritive' and 'integrative' authority, both can be a feature of position or personal authority. Nutritive authority is used *for* or on behalf of another and the latter *with* another. For example, one who fosters a collaborative form of government is exercising an integrative quality; one who acts for the welfare of another

51   See Gordon Lawrence (1989) *Social Dreaming for the Management of Change: A Programme of Dialogues.* London: Grubb Institute.

person, but without their involvement, is using nutritive authority.[52] The paternalistic control of the colonial Fijian government was nutritive, but ultimately a failure, while Ganey's authority was integrative with outstandingly successful consequences for human growth.

Subsidiarity and accountability

The principle of subsidiarity, as explained in Chapter 4, means that whatever people are able to do for themselves ought not to be removed from their competence and taken over by other people. Decisions should not be made at higher levels if they can be effectively made lower down. However, the formal leader will ensure that roles and boundaries for team members are clarified so that people do not needlessly interfere in what others are delegated to do. If the boundaries of respective competencies are smudged, all kinds of quite unnecessary tensions and conflicts will emerge, draining energy inwards that should be directed outwards to the realization of the team's mission. Subsidiarity also means that leaders must guard these boundaries and call people to be accountable in their roles. One of the major problems in healthcare institutions has been the failure to clarify the complementary roles of clinicians and managers. As described in Chapter 3, this has caused significant frustration to all concerned, with negative consequences for the safety and welfare of patients. The neglect of role clarification and accountability has seriously contributed to the poisonous cultures of bullying in healthcare (see Chapter 4). An example of what happens when the principle of subsidiarity in healthcare is overlooked is evident in New South Wales, Australia. The decision was made to centralize financial and administrative decision-making in the Department of Health. The links between hospitals and local communities were broken and eight new administrative structures were established under the Department of Health. It was overall a costly financial and human failure. The new structures were too big for local people to relate to; and the decision-makers were too remote from the people affected by these decisions, namely 'the managers and clincians working at the hospital and unit level'.[53]

---

52   See Rollo May (1972) *Power and Innocence*. New York: Norton, pp.105–109.
53   Garling 2008b, p.31.

Courage and imagination

True leaders are courageous and imaginative people. They are prepared to take risks to achieve their goals, just as my mother did every time she rode her bicycle without lights to see a sick person. My mother was so pained by the gap between the founding values of healthcare and the reality that she imaginatively and creatively aimed to bridge the gap through carefully devised strategies. Imagination is the ability to picture a world beyond what we accept as the status quo. It is the capacity to hold freely what the world assumes and to venture into alternative outlines of reality, which is only hinted at. The role of the paramodern leader is to foster a subversion of reality that persistently undermines the ordinary. The stark fact is that many healthcare institutions never succeed in reinventing themselves because people lack the courage and imagination to challenge deeply held assumptions about existing strategies and processes and, in response, to think and act in fundamentally altered ways. Rather, most persist doing the same old things in superficially changed ways – practices that are quite inadequate for survival and growth in contemporary healthcare circumstances.[54] There must be a collaborative willingness to let cherished structures and processes die when they no longer serve the mission. Peter Drucker warned that few 'service institutions attempt to think through the changed circumstances in which they operate.' He writes that there 'is the need for a systematic withdrawal of resources of money, but above all, of people – from yesterday's efforts.'[55] For this to happen, courage and imagination are essential.

New belongs elsewhere

A basic assumption in this chapter is that positive innovation in healthcare can only take place in an environment in which growth can occur. It requires a cultural climate, based on the values of paramodernity, in which members can view one another as resources rather than competitors or judges according to the ethos of modernity. It requires a climate of openness and mutual support in which differences are confronted and worked through, and in

54   Edgar H. Schein, interviewed by Coutu 2002, p.100.
55   Peter Drucker (1982) *Managing in Turbulent Times*. London: Pan Books, p.46.

which feedback on performance is a mutual responsibility among members so that all can learn to contribute more. As explained, resistance to cultural change is to some degree natural and inevitable (see Chapter 1). Yet resistance can become so entrenched that creative leaders are in danger of becoming emotionally exhausted by their efforts to challenge the status quo. It is at this point that the guideline 'the new belongs elsewhere' needs to be evoked. That is, structures and lines of accountability are built to shield creative persons from undue interference from outsiders.[56] This does not mean that innovative people are to be protected from all conflict, because creativity is born of tension, passion and conflict. It is rather a question of protecting creative people from negative conflict, that is, conflict that does not serve the mission. An analogy with the human body helps to explain the relevance of the guideline, 'the new belongs elsewhere'. In coronary artery disease progressive obstruction in arteries restricts the blood flow to the heart; if the problem is left unchecked, death is inevitable. Because the welfare of the total body has priority, surgeons take healthy veins from other parts of the body and turn them upside down to make them into arteries that bypass the diseased arteries. The bypass operation, through the use of 'new structures', that is, the grafted healthy veins, allows the patient to be, as it were, 'refounded'.

CASE STUDY: REFOUNDING

The board of management of a hospital, supported by the trustees, accepted the plan of a heart surgeon to establish a research unit. The surgeon felt the unit could be attached to an existing vascular research department, but the board disagreed. Being concerned that unnecessary time and energy of a specialist would be lost in obtaining the research department's approval and support to begin and continue the venture, the board decided to establish the unit as a separate entity directly responsible to itself. This was done and the unit was quickly established and continues to flourish today.[57]

---

56   See Peter Drucker (1986) *Innovation and Entrepreneurship: Practice and Principles.* New York: Harper & Row, pp.161–164.

57   See Arbuckle 2000, pp.218–219.

Here, the board formulated clear lines of authority and accountability. The reason for its success was that outsiders knew they could not interfere. The project was explained to other departments, and any significant interaction with the heart unit was required to go through the board's representative. The specialist was instructed to keep the board regularly informed of the unit's progress; the board agreed to inform the hospital and wider community about the unit. In this way the surgeon and fellow researchers were freed to use their talents and energies directly for the project.

Refounding

Paramodern leaders are inspired by the values of the founding mythology, but at the same time, they are deeply pained by the gap between those values and the world in which they live. They know that to lose the founding story is to lose direction and the energy for action. They therefore draw other people, as my mother did, to share their inspiration and pain in order that together they can creatively find ways to build bridges across the gulf separating the founding mythology from contemporary realities. Collaborators recognize that their own talents and journey in life can fit into the narrative of the organization in a mutually advantageous way.[58] In Guideline 6, Chapter 1, it was explained that creative action requires the radical breakdown of the cultural status quo. Paramodern leaders take advantage of existing organizational chaos or even create it in order that refounding can occur. As Schein wrote, if an organization 'is to change its culture, it must be led by someone who can, in effect, break the tyranny of the old culture'.[59] Chaos is viewed as necessary and positive, the opportunity to keep creating radically new ways of acting in order to respond to constantly changing needs. This is contrary to the traditional wisdom of people who are devoted to modernity's view of what leaders should do; for them, the primary task of healthcare leaders is to make decisions that foster and maintain orderly relationships.[60] For them, whatever is confusing,

---

58   See MacLeod and Clarke 2009, p.75.
59   Schein 1985, p.321.
60   See McDaniel 1997.

disorderly, or chaotic is 'unnatural', to be considered dangerous to the survival of the organization.

This process of collaboratively bridging the gap in chaotic situations is called refounding, that is, a process of reowning the founding values of healthcare and innovatively applying them to contemporary healthcare issues and going to the very roots of problems. An analogy will help to explain the radical difference between refounding and renewing. If my car has a puncture, I either repair it, replace it with the spare tyre or buy a new one so that I can restore the vehicle to its primary task of getting me from A to B. If I choose any of these options, I become involved in *renewing* the car. But to 'refound the car', however, I would need to invent a form of transport that is quite significantly different, for example, invent a hovercraft that has no wheels and so does not get punctures. A contemporary example from the retailing industry further illustrates the distinction between renewal and refounding. Following the initial impact of online shopping at the beginning of this century most bricks-and-mortar shops, such as Walmart and Target, have made only renewal or superficial changes to their business model. Ostrich-like, they have tried to ignore the huge consequences of online shopping; they are failing to make radical changes to their ways of doing business and attracting customers. Consequently without refounding many retail shops now risk extinction. To continue these bricks-and-mortar stores need enormous imagination and creativity under the direction of skilled and courageous leadership, not the mere modifications of existing processes. Unless they are prepared for refounding we will see an increasing number of failures among once-flourishing companies. Witness the sudden demise of the now extinct worldwide bookshop chain of Borders.[61]

Certainly, in healthcare, we need both processes, that is, renewal and refounding, but the refounding is by far the more difficult and fraught with the inevitable tensions associated with culture change. For example, in the public hospitals of New South Wales the challenge was to develop a 'new model of teamwork...to replace the old and independent "silos" of professional care'.[62] Tinkering

---

61 See 'Retailers and the internet: Clicks and bricks.' (2012) *The Economist* (25 February), 14–15.
62 Garling 2008b, p.4.

with the symptoms of the schism-like divide between various levels of management, different 'tribes' of clinicians, medical clinicians and managers, will not solve the problem (see Chapter 3). Rather, leaders are required who can go to penetrate to the roots of the problem and develop appropriate collaborative teamwork.

Examples of refounding

- Jean Vanier, Canadian philosopher and humanitarian, is the founder of 150 communities for people with severe developmental disabilities. While a doctoral student in Paris in the mid-1960s he became painfully aware of how these individuals were locked away from society, often in very inhuman conditions. Believing that such people can, in fact, play a full role in society if only society would allow them, he formed small outward-facing communities where people with and without disabilities could share life, affirming one another's unique values and gifts. In so doing, he has refounded the whole approach to society's relationship to people with developmental disabilities based on values of compassion, empathy, dialogue and mutuality.[63]

- Dame Cecily Saunders is another refounding person in healthcare. As Western medicine focused on the biomedical model, it lost its caring touch. This was particularly evident in the approach to the dying, who increasingly found themselves to be unwelcome anomalies in the system of high technology medicine (see Chapter 2). Recognizing this, Saunders refounded care of the dying through the creation of what has become the contemporary worldwide hospice and palliative care movement. Care of the dying should address not only the medical concerns of patients, but also their emotional and spiritual needs. She created a medical speciality which uses skills based on the most up-to-date scientific knowledge, while, at the same time, recognizing the importance of a truly caring attitude and approach. At the heart of the hospice movement is a philosophy that embraces a network of values and attitudes

---

63   See Kathryn Spink (2006) *The Miracle, The Message, The Story: Jean Vanier.* London: Darton, Longman and Todd.

that tries to lessen the indignities of dying so as to maximize the human potential of dying people and their families.[64]

○ In New South Wales, Australia, in 2008 it was found that the detection and management of deterioration in a patient's condition by hospital staff could be problematic, especially where the difficulties developed overnight when patients were under the care of junior clinicians who might lack the experience to deal with them or were hesitant to disturb the consultant.[65] The Department of Health, on the initiative of the state's Clinical Excellence Commission, introduced a programme ('Between the Flags')[66] the following year that provided a standardized system for clinicians to recognize and respond to patients who were clinically deteriorating. A detailed evaluation in 2010 found that the programme had become widely successful. In particular, junior staff members indicated that the programme empowered them 'to advocate for a patient by creating a systematic approach to identifying and following up "at risk" patients'.[67] The main reasons for the success of the programme were: committed and skilled leadership, a thorough educational programme for clinicians and the clarity of the warning signs of deterioration and the clearly stated step-by-step responses required of clinicians.[68] In a review of the programme, it was found that 'it has reduced the number of adverse outcomes such as cardiac arrests and has provided a constructive framework for nursing staff to engage with junior medical officers'.[69] It has proved that it is possible for the Department of Health and Clinical Excellence

---

64   See Cecily Saunders (1997) 'Hospices Worldwide: A Mission Statement.' In Cecily Saunders and Robert Kastenbaum (eds) *Hospice Care on the International Scene*. New York: Springer, pp.3–12.

65   See Garling 2008b, p.25.

66   The title of the programme, 'Between the Flags', is particularly appropriate for Australians. On Australian beaches people are advised for their safety to swim only between the two flags where lifeguards patrol.

67   NSW Independent Panel (2011) *Final Progress Report on the Implementation of the Government's Response to the Special Commission of Inquiry into Acute Care Services in NSW Hospitals* (July 2011). Sydney: NSW Independent Panel, p.13.

68   Ibid.

69   NSW Independent Panel 2010a, p.30.

Commission to collaborate constructively.[70] This is an excellent example of refounding because the champions of the change process, out of respect for the welfare of patients and concern for junior clinicians, went to the heart of the problem: the failure to provide clear and accountable guidelines for detecting signs of deterioration and an appropriate educational programme for clinicians in the use of the guidelines.

Storytelling

When I interviewed Cecily Saunders in 1989 at St Christopher's Hospice, London, the world's first purpose-built hospice, I asked her why she had started the hospice movement. She simply responded by retelling a very personal and inspiring story. In 1948, she fell in love with a patient dying of cancer, David Tasma, a Polish-Jewish refugee who, having survived the Warsaw ghetto, made a living as a waiter. It was this experience of caring that moved her to think about establishing the hospice movement. When David died he left £500 for, as he said, 'a window in your home', that would symbolically represent the hospice movement that Cecily had begun to dream about establishing. It took 11 years before the project came to fruition. As I listened to her recounting the founding of the hospice movement, I felt I was back with her in 1948 caring for David Tasma. I could feel something of the pain she had experienced as she reflected on the sterility of the biomedical model in the presence of a dying person. For me, the interview was a vivid, intensely uplifting experience. I left her company feeling energized and further committed myself to the task of holistic healthcare. I had a similar experience when interviewing Jean Vanier, listening to his pain of hearing people with learning disabilities who were marginalized by society, often drugged to keep them quiet and less annoying to 'normal' people. He talked to me of his experience with Raphael and Philippe, the two people with developmental disabilities who joined him in the first L'Arche community in Paris, of how hard it was to begin 'to listen to' rather than 'wanting all the time to do things for'.

Stories can empathetically tell people who they are, where they come from, what is good or bad for them and the way they are

---

70   Ibid., p.31.

to organize themselves and maintain their sense of unique identity in a challenging world. Stories can give people a sense of energy and direction. Merely rational arguments about the way the world is changing and why identity is so important sound flat and inane. In abstract thinking, listeners are rarely moved to any magic world of identity, a conceptual 'elsewhere' that they can recognize, or in which they feel comfortable. On the other hand, stories such as those that recount the founding of a nation or an organization are the emotional glue that can bind people together at the deepest level of their collective being (see Chapter 1).[71] However, they have this impact only when they are skilfully retold, especially in times of uncertainty and tumultuous change. Today, when hospice or L'Arche people are asked to explain these movements, they repeat these stories or narratives that ultimately have their roots in the original founding story of healthcare.

This emphasis on storytelling does not downplay the importance of abstract thinking and analysis. Storytelling can supplement analytical thinking by encouraging people to imagine new angles of a complex issue. Abstract analysis is easier to grasp when viewed through the lens of a suitably selected incident or narrative of another person's life journey.[72] Stephen Denning, Program Director of Knowledge Management, The World Bank, began his book on storytelling for organizational change in the following personal way:

> Why storytelling? Nothing else worked. Charts left listeners bemused. Prose remained unread. Dialogue was just too laborious and slow. Time after time, when faced with the task of persuading a group of managers…in a large organization to get enthusiastic about a major change, I found that storytelling was the only thing that worked.[73]

---

71 See Herminia Ibarra and Kent Lineback (2005) 'What's your story? Managing yourself.' *Harvard Business Review 83*, 1, 65–71; Michael Kaye (1996) *Myth-Makers and Story-Tellers*. Sydney: Business and Professional Publishing.

72 See Stephen Denning (2001) *The Springboard: How Storytelling Ignites Action in Knowledge-Era Organizations*. Boston, MA: Butterworth-Heinemann, p.xvii.

73 Ibid., p.xiii. Denning is currently Senior Fellow at the James MacGregor Burns Leadership Academy, University of Maryland, USA. John Kotter, the award-winning professor at Harvard Business School, and Holger Rathgeber, have written a fable in book form in order to teach readers about the art of leadership. See John Kotter and Holger Rothgeber (2006) *Our Iceberg is Melting: Changing and Succeeding under Any Conditions*. London: Macmillan.

There are several types of storytelling. People may fashion their identity by recounting their own experiences for the first time, or they may turn to the narratives of others as models to guide them. Visionaries like Martin Luther King, Jr and Nelson Mandela provide road maps through darkness to light. There are also fictional stories from which readers and listeners are enabled to articulate their own sense of sadness and hope. For example, the great novelist J.R.R. Tolkien wrote that fictional stories are 'prophylactic against loss' in a way which permits the loss to be named. It is through the quasi-experience of loss which fiction evokes, that listeners and readers are able to gain a certain therapeutic permission to reconnect with truths from which they may be sheltered in daily life.[74] Tolkein wrote profoundly on this point:

> Probably every writer making a secondary world, a fantasy, every sub-creator…hopes that the peculiar qualities of this secondary world are derived from Reality, or are flowing into it…The peculiar quality of the 'joy' in successful Fantasy can thus be explained as a sudden glimpse of the underlying reality or truth. It is not only a 'consolation' for the sorrow of this world, but a satisfaction, and an answer to the question, 'Is it true?'[75]

Then there are springboard stories which communicate new ideas in ways that help people to understand their complexity and be encouraged to overcome their resistance to change. The stories bypass the normal defences and engage people's feelings. In this way the storyteller is so able to engage listeners so that they see that they themselves can act in a similar way to change their environment.[76]

CASE STUDY: STORYTELLING

When I first began to consult as an applied anthropologist to public and non-profit healthcare systems about paramodern leadership I made a serious mistake. I began with lectures and then invited participants to respond to questions based on what I had been saying, but I quickly discovered that this top-down approach did not work. Instead, in an interactive way, I invited people to identify public, operative residual

---

74   See Richard Kearney (2002) *On Stories*. London: Routledge, p.26.
75   J.R.R. Tolkein (1968) *The Tolkein Reader*. Princeton, NJ: Princeton University Press, p.88.
76   See Denning 2001, p.xv.

myths in their cultural worlds. I would then explain the Good Samaritan parable, as the founding myth of healthcare, inviting participants to identify how their own behaviour and the culture of their institution or department conformed or not to the values in the story. The Good Samaritan parable became a catalyst or springboard story for animated storytelling by participants. One participant summarized the reactions of many: 'For the first time I have had the chance to reflect on why I want to work in this system. The values of the parable are what I want to see alive in my hospital culture and I will continue to do my best to contribute to this culture.' Participants became so involved and energized that it was difficult to bring the sessions to closure. On other occasions, collaborative groups set themselves practical projects based on the values and to be completed within definite time limits. They would regularly inform others of the progress of these projects, illustrating, in story form, how the projects related to the founding values of healthcare.

Listening and reflecting

Paramodern leaders are listening people who want to understand what others feel and think. Nothing is more conducive to building trust in an institution than the willingness of leaders to listen, that is, the openness to hear the appealing and the unappealing, the familiar and the unfamiliar. Yet to listen to others leaders must first be prepared to listen to themselves – their inner fears, motives, intuitions. This requires periods of stillness and silence. In the executive wing of one large healthcare system, the CEO set aside a well-designed 'room of contemplation' where staff could go and spend time just to think, to remove themselves from the pressures of the desks. It was well patronized and much appreciated by busy executives. Psychoanalyst Wilfred Bion strongly advised his colleagues to admit at times in their clinical work that they did not know the answers to the problems confronting them. He tells them to sit in the darkness of *not-knowing*:

> Discard your memory; discard the future tense of your desire...to leave a space for a new idea... Instead of trying to bring a brilliant, intelligent, knowledgeable light to bear on obscure problems, I suggest we bring to bear a diminution of the light – a penetrating

beam of darkness. Thus, a very faint light would become visible in maximum conditions of darkness.[77]

To sit in the darkness/chaos of 'not-knowing', without distractions and the busyness of daily life, expecting no immediate insights, is paradoxically the way to new insights and self-knowledge.

Thinking big/thinking small

Paramodern leaders are consultative people. Culture is primarily about maintaining order, not change (see Chapter 1, Guidelines 2, 3, 7). Unless people are duly consulted and feel the need for change, they will resist change. Consultation takes time, but it will ensure that culture change occurs and is sustained. A paramodern leader will also first focus their energy on small groups which then become models for others to observe and follow. The leader also recognizes the wisdom of the guideline: 'To think big in change, think small!' The vision can be huge, but the steps to realize this vision need to be clearly visible and realizable. People will lose interest, develop resistance, if they are unable to see that each achieved step in a project is concretely related to the overall vision.

Summary

- There is much confusion about the meaning of leadership in policy documents on healthcare. It is often made synonymous with management. They have different but complementary roles: the manager emphasizes systems and structures, the leader focuses on people and culture; the manager maintains the status quo, the leader questions it; the manager fosters an atmosphere of control, the leader inspires people to be creative.

- Leaders, who are committed to the reform of healthcare systems, must be able, *inter alia,* to form doctors into teams, 'measure their performance not by how much they do but by how their patients fare; deftly apply financial and behavioral

---

77   Wilfred Bion, as cited by Patrick J. Casement (1991) *Learning from the Patient.* New York: Guilford Press, p.358.

incentives',[78] and to do this they must be able to demolish obstructive cultures. This means that the task of leadership in healthcare should be to foster a collaborative or participative atmosphere in which trust and mutuality exist as the prerequisites for creative action or strategies for cultural change. Leaders must constantly be seeking ways of working collaboratively in unpredictable environments, such as is the case in healthcare, rather than becoming involved in useless efforts to make things less unpredictable. Only in this way can cultural resistances to change be managed.[79] This is paramodern leadership.

○ Paramodern leadership is based on neither a cult of individualism nor the exaltation of a hierarchical, self-centred status system. Paramodern leaders foster collaborative planning and action based on a commonly agreed mission, vision and values that, in this case, have their origin in the founding story of Western healthcare, namely the Good Samaritan parable.

○ When they meet excessive resistance to change, paramodern leaders adopt the guideline 'the new belongs elsewhere', that is, they develop structures of authority and accountability to protect creative people from undue and exhausting interference. Demonstrated successes by these innovators is the best way to attract the majority of people to examine new ways of working together.

○ Paramodern leaders are uncomfortable colleagues as they relentlessly question conventional wisdom for the sake of the mission. Any organization that domesticates its rebels has acquired its peace, but it has lost its future. Inspired by the memory of the founding mythology and values of healthcare, leaders are able to lead cultural change creatively and in significant ways relevant to contemporary needs.

○ One of the most important and neglected task for a paramodern leader is to offer space to people and cultures to grieve over what has died or is no longer relevant. When one accepts the reality of loss, with its pain and anger, and allows it to

---

78   See Lee 2010, p.53.
79   See Paul Bate (1994) *Strategies for Cultural Change*. Oxford: Butterworth-Heinemann, p.147.

pass, then the new reality has room to enter. If losses are not acknowledged they remain to haunt us, trapping people and cultures unwittingly in the past.

○ It has been said that in healthcare as in other organizations 'mergers and acquisitions can turn otherwise rational executives into emotional wrecks and transform well-meaning managers into seeming monsters'.[80] Chapter 6 argues that one significant cause of this is the failure to appreciate the importance of the cultural factors in mergers.

Strategic implications
Policies

○ Financial pressures and technological discoveries in the field and healthcare are calling for changes in healthcare cultures at an ever-increasing rate. These pressures and discoveries demand not just incremental organizational changes, but at times radical shifts in thinking and action. Yet organizational cultures are resistant to changes (see Chapter 1); people and cultures cannot be changed simply by a management decree or by merely rearranging the structures. Therefore, for change to be effective and in line with the foundational values of healthcare, collaborative and innovative leaders must be in place at all institutional levels.

Implementation

○ Since research shows it takes on average 60 ideas before one innovation is initiated,[81] the most practical course a manager can take to encourage leadership and creativity in healthcare is to foster a culture of trust and ease of communication. The more that trust and openness are encouraged, the more

---

80 Philip H. Mirvis and Mitchell Lee Marks (1992) *Managing the Merger: Making it Work.* Paramus, NJ: Prentice Hall, p.xvii.

81 See Simon Majaro (1995) 'Creativity in the Search for Strategy.' In Stuart Crainer (ed.) *The Financial Times Handbook of Management.* London: Pitman Publishing, p.165.

people are willing to articulate their ideas for evaluation and experimentation.

○ Leaders of cultural change in this area will recognize the need to constantly clarify the mission and values of their institutions as changes occur, but in ways that involve staff members (see Chapter 1); this will mean giving people the space to align their personal values with the foundational values of healthcare.

○ Because the challenges facing the reform of healthcare institutions are so daunting, people can fatalistically feel there is nothing they can do. Leaders of cultural change, however, know that one person can still make a difference. Hence, in order to empower people to assume a leadership role in cultural change, it is important that managers identify examples of successful change-agents from the past and the present and encourage their stories to be told. Storytelling, as explained above, brings abstract ideas and values down to earth and demonstrates that people individually and collaboratively can lead cultural change in healthcare.

○ Managers need to identify, support and publicly congratulate people in their institutions who show collaborative and creative leadership that is based on the foundational values of healthcare; this may mean establishing structures that protect the innovators from wearying interference from the surrounding organizational culture.

CHAPTER 6

Leading Mergers in Healthcare
Cultural Processes

They [mergers] are, like second marriages, a triumph of hope over experience. A stream of studies has shown that corporate mergers have even higher failure rates than the liaisons of Hollywood stars.

(Chris Anderson et al.)[1]

Let sorrow lend me words, and words express
The manner of my pity-wanting pain.

(William Shakespeare)[2]

This chapter explains:

○ that the most common reasons for the high failure rate of mergers in healthcare and elsewhere are the poverty of leadership and the failure to appreciate the cultural issues involved before, during and after a merger

○ that the word 'merger' is used in many different senses, but common to all is that some degree of cultural change is involved

○ that appropriate communication, led by executives as 'ritual leaders', is crucial for the success of a merger of organizational cultures

○ that traditional peoples teach us that merging of cultures is a rite of passage or initiation to a new mythology and values through three stages: separation, *liminality* and re-entry. Each stage contains specific communication needs.

---

1   Chris Anderson *et al.* (2000) *Making Mergers Work*. London: The Economist, p.3.
2   William Shakespeare, *Sonnets*, no. cxi.

The term 'merger' is commonly used to cover such organizational changes as joint ventures, strategic alliances, networks, acquisitions, partnerships or restructuring.[3] Strictly speaking it refers to the process whereby organizations dialogue as equals, with the intention of producing a single new entity with its own culture, frequently with a new name. Whether the term is used loosely or strictly, however, some degree of cultural change is required.

In the United States the number of hospital mergers continues to grow. In 1979 only 31 per cent of hospitals were part of a wider hospital system but by 2001 the figure had risen to 50 per cent. Today almost 60 per cent of all hospitals are part of systems, and it is predicted that by 2015 stand-alone community hospitals will cease to exist.[4] The assumption is that mergers will lead to more capital being available for development, better management and more influence when negotiating treatment prices with health insurers. In England an increase in mergers of hospitals is anticipated as part of the overall reform of the NHS.

Unfortunately, the history of organizational mergers is a dismal one. They are often undertaken for the best of reasons, only for the organizations to discover that their hopes of significant success is unrealized. In the early 1990s it was estimated that, in the United States, between two-thirds and three-fourths of all corporate mergers and acquisitions fail,[5] up to one-third collapse within five years 'and as many as 80% never live up to full expectations'.[6] Healthcare mergers are no exception; in the early 1990s some 75 per cent had not succeeded or at best had not reached their planned potential, and the pattern continues today.[7] A 2010 report on mergers in the NHS is gloomy: it is estimated that a success rate of more than 25 to 30 per cent would be optimistic.[8] Mergers have come to be associated with lowered morale, job dissatisfaction, unproductive behaviour,

3   See Maria Goddard and Brian Ferguson (1997) *Mergers in NHS: Made in Heaven or Marriages of Convenience.* London: Nuffield Trust, pp.13–14; Arbuckle 2000, pp.271–303.

4   See Michael Rowan (2011) 'Amid promise and peril, hold mission high.' *Health Progress 92,* 2, 12.

5   See Mirvis and Marks 1992, p.vii.

6   See Ernst & Young and Brian Miller (eds) (1994) *Mergers and Acquisitions: Back-to-Basics Techniques for the 90s,* 2nd edn. New York: John Wiley, p.230.

7   See Janet Field and Edward Peck (2003) 'Mergers and acquisitions in the private sector: What are the lessons for health and social services?' *Social Policy and Administration 37,* 7, 742–755.

8   See NHS Confederation (2010) *Lessons from the History of Reorganisation.* London: NHS Confederation, pp.2, 4–5.

sabotage, petty theft, absenteeism and increased labour turnover, strikes and accident rates, rather than with increased profitability.[9] Other dysfunctional effects include 'a loss of focus on services, delays in service improvements and a difficulty in transferring good practice within the merged organisation'.[10] Two observers bluntly concluded that mergers 'can turn otherwise rational executives into emotional wrecks and transform well-meaning managers into seeming monsters'.[11] Failures can be measured in financial terms, but it is impossible to assess the human suffering that these collapses cause.

The poverty of leadership and the failure to appreciate the cultural issues involved before, during and after are the two most common interconnected reasons given for the high failure rate of mergers.[12] What Jill Sherer concluded in her review of hospital mergers in the early 1990s remains relevant today: 'Studies show that as many as 75% of hospital-hospital mergers are unsuccessful when issues surrounding corporate culture are ignored.'[13] It is relatively straightforward to decide optimistically on a plan for structural changes, but if cultural issues are ignored, no amount of administrative planning will produce positive results. Another observer also concluded that cultural factors are the 'significant largest cause of the lack of projected performance, departure of key executives, and time-consuming conflicts'[14] in mergers. Among other deficiencies, leaders commonly fail to clarify precisely the purpose of a merger.[15] One observer of healthcare mergers in the United States concluded that: 'Too often the board's decision-making process could be characterized as "aim, fire, ready or not." Boards frequently…miss a vital first step: probing in-depth their core values and their needs for a strategic partner.'[16] If people fail to ask the question 'Why merge?', it is scarcely surprising that they also neglect the cultural factors that

9   Ibid., p.5; George Meeks (1977) *Disappointing Marriages: A Study of the Gains from Mergers.* Cambridge: Cambridge University Press; Sue Cartwright and Cary L. Cooper (1993) 'The psychological impact of merger and acquisition on the individual.' *Human Relations 46*, 3, 327–329.

10   NHS Confederation 2010, 2.

11   Mirvis and Mitchell 1992, p.xvii.

12   See Schein 1985, p.29.

13   Jill Sherer (1994) 'Corporate cultures.' *Hospitals and Health Networks* (5 May), 19–22.

14   Ernst & Young and Miller 1994, p.230.

15   See NHS Confederation 2010, p.7.

16   Barry S. Bader (1977) 'Look before you leap: Boards need to ask "why?" before merging or affiliating.' *Trustee 50*, 3, 20.

accompany the process of merging. In brief, mergers have a chance to succeed *if* the purpose is first clarified, and *if* leaders are prepared to acknowledge throughout the process the critical importance of the cultural factors involved. Too much emphasis is given to hoped-for financial benefits in the planning of a merger, neglecting cultural issues. This is a recipe for disaster. Daryl Conner correctly observed that the difficulties with mergers and acquisitions primarily come from 'a misalignment of two cultures and are compounded by a lack of skill for cultural management on both sides'.[17] The fact that, in proposed mergers, 'the tools for assessing cultural differences are still relatively crude',[18] scarcely helps.

In the light of the central importance of cultural issues in mergers and the frequent lack of clarity regarding them, the following are practical interconnected guidelines to assist people committed to leading mergers in healthcare.

Practical guidelines

Guideline 1: Before proceeding with a merger leaders must clarify its purpose and undertake a process of 'due diligence' that includes an assessment of cultural compatibility

If the purpose is fuzzy, unnecessary chaos will result and the merger will inevitably fail. 'Due diligence', the business assessment of a proposed merger, must include an evaluation of cultural compatibility. If values in the two organizations are fundamentally similar, then the merger has a good chance of succeeding. For an effective evaluation of cultural compatibility it is not sufficient to compare mission statements and written descriptions of structural organizational systems. These statements and systems could coincide perfectly but their implementation could in practice radically differ. Hence, to assess the values of an organizational culture it will be necessary to *observe*, for example, *how* decisions are really made, whether or not people are committed to teamwork, their openness to change and the level of employee satisfaction. This type of review requires

---

17 Daryl R. Conner (1993) *Managing at the Speed of Change.* New York: Villard Books, p.174.
18 Schein 1985, p.36.

skill and time, but if the merger proceeds without this process, then disasters are bound to result.[19]

By way of summary, it is important to repeat this warning. It is my experience that on paper the administrative structures and mission statements can be perfectly aligned, while the lived mythologies and values of the institutions remain radically different. If this is the case, the efforts to merge the institutions will be extremely costly in human and financial terms, with little chance of a successful merger. This point will be further explained in Guideline 2.

Guideline 2: In assessing cultural compatibility it is essential for leaders to recognize the three types of founding myths in organizations – the public, operational and residual. The practical recognition of the differences between them will contribute to the success of a merger

It is my experience that mergers often fail simply because no one recognizes the fundamental differences of the founding myths of the organizational cultures to be merged. For example, on paper it may immediately seem logical for two, geographically close, non-profit hospitals in the United States to merge in order to achieve the benefits of integrated delivery and to be able to compete successfully with a newly established hospital nearby. Everything, it could be said, favours the merger, because even their mission statements are very similar. Why should the trustees hesitate? The answer is a cultural one. The founding myths of the two hospitals, despite the similarities of their mission statements, are likely to be radically different. Failure to investigate these founding myths could well lead to disaster. Why might this be so? As explained in Chapter 1, we must distinguish three types of myth: public, operative and residual. A public myth is a set of stated ideals, such as those contained in vision and mission statements, that people publicly commit themselves to strive to implement. It is relatively easy to formulate a public myth. This myth becomes an operational myth only when people actually put the public myth into practice. In-built cultural resistances can, however, make this a difficult, if not an impossible, task. Residual

---

19   See Stephen J. Wall and Shannon Rye Wall (2000) *The Morning After: Making Corporate Mergers Work after the Deal is Sealed*. Cambridge, MA: Perseus, pp.75–97.

myths within the cultures to be merged lurk beneath the surface and can re-emerge when people least expect. In our hypothetical example, the fact that the two hospitals have existed close by for a long time means that they have inevitably been competing for patients. Their organizational cultures would have become distrustful of each other, reinforced by memories of negative incidents in the past. These suspicions would continue to lurk beneath the surface as residual myths; unless these disruptive myths are surfaced and acknowledged they would eventually return and destroy the desired collaboration between the two hospitals through a merger.

Guideline 3: The founding mythologies of non-profit and for-profit healthcare services are fundamentally different[20]

Particularly in the United States, for-profit organizations are increasingly interested in acquiring existing non-profit healthcare services. However, the cultures are radically different. A non-profit will do everything it can to maintain its mission of holistic healthcare and its concern for people on the margins of society. A for-profit, on the other hand, must primarily focus on providing good financial returns to its investors.[21]

Guideline 4: Leaders must clarify and continually communicate the purpose of a merger

Throughout the merging process it is almost impossible for leaders to communicate excessively to all concerned. Despite the time involved, leaders, or their carefully trained delegates, must make themselves visible and available to all employees affected by the merger. Rumours and gossip circulating among staff members about aspects of the mergers can have devastating negative consequences, but these can be minimized through frequent and accurate information.[22]

---

20 See Arbuckle 2000, pp.282–287.
21 See Amata Miller (1996) 'Merging with for-profits: Flawed strategies.' *Health Progress* 77, 4, 16.
22 See Ernst & Young and Miller 1994, pp.241–243.

CASE STUDY: LEICESTER ROYAL INFIRMARY NATIONAL HEALTH SERVICE

Radical structural changes were needed to improve the quality and efficiency of the Leicester Royal Infirmary NHS, England, a large, complex, teaching hospital serving around 500,000 patients annually. Because this necessitated the merging of its internal processes, substantial cultural readjustments were necessary. The following lessons emerged from this successful venture:[23]

- Those responsible for leading the merger must themselves be united as a team and committed to building a task-oriented culture; they are to model what the entire system is to be.

- It is necessary to spend considerable time and energy training managers at all levels for their new roles; the involvement of 'clinical colleagues in the development of managerial and supervisory roles cannot be underestimated... Senior managers have a critical role [as they] must protect the organisation as it reinvents itself.'[24]

- Throughout the merging process, creative cultural change agents are to be identified and supported; one of the best ways to achieve the support of the majority of staff members is to point to the positive effects of their leadership.

- There is a need to continue to communicate clearly and widely to the whole system the progress of the merger, pointing out how this is in line with the vision and mission of the merger.

Guideline 5: Recognize that the process of in-depth organizational cultural change following formal mergers is bound to be slow and hesitant

This guideline is fully explained in Chapter 1, Guideline 7. Resistance comes from fear of the unknown. As Charles Handy warned, organizational cultures contemplating a merger are 'stuck with their past...their traditions. These things take years if not decades to change.'[25] Implementers of mergers, who are insensitive

---

23   See Oram and Wellins 1995, pp.33–42.
24   Ibid., pp.129, 170.
25   Charles Handy (1985) *Understanding Voluntary Organizations*. London: Penguin, p.95.

to the difficulties of culture change and people's feelings, are apt to become more dogmatic and imperious in their commands to staff. This causes staff morale to drop further and their resistance to change increases. This, in turn, generates increasing anger and impatience in managers, further reinforcing the cycle of resistance. In summary, when change challenges a culture it is the culture that most commonly wins. Unless the conflicting feelings that the merger process evokes can be surfaced and sensitively confronted by leaders, they will linger on and hold back the merging process. But we must not underestimate how difficult this is. I commonly find that sensitive cultural leadership is a rare gift. If people are oblivious of the power of culture in their own lives they are bound to be unconscious of its importance for other people. Anthropologist Edward Hall correctly observed that a culture 'hides most effectively from its own participants'. To be sensitively aware of one's own culture 'is an achievement of gargantuan proportions for anyone'.[26]

Guideline 6: In the process of merging cultures, not just individuals experience grief

Grief describes the sadness, sorrow, confusion, even guilt, that can emerge when individuals suffer loss. C.S. Lewis described the frightening power of grief he experienced following the death of his wife: 'No one told me that grief felt so like fear. I am not afraid, but the sensation is like being afraid. The same fluttering in the stomach, the same restlessness, the yawning.'[27] However, cultures, not just individuals, experience grief over loss with the accompanying feelings of anger, despair and helplessness. One has but to recall the nationwide grief in the United States after the tragic terrorist assault in New York in 2001, the national feeling of loss in Britain following the later terrorist attack in London that killed 52 people and, more recently, the collective grief that followed the massive earthquakes in New Zealand and Japan. The grief transcended the anguish of individuals but also affected them at the same time. The following example illustrates a similar experience in a hospital culture when confronted with dramatic loss.

---

26   Hall 1959, p.30.
27   C.S. Lewis (1961) *A Grief Observed*. London: Faber & Faber, p.7.

CASE STUDY: HOSPITAL CLOSURE AND COLLECTIVE GRIEF

In Australia a state government suddenly and unexpectedly announced in the early morning news that an historic and well-loved central-city public hospital was to close and its services were to be transferred to an existing hospital in a distant suburb. A short time later, I walked into the hospital's foyer and immediately felt the collective shock. Even if I had not known of the decision, I would have felt the collective grief that affected not just the staff, but also the patients. As I walked through the foyer into other parts of the hospital, I could feel people's anger, sadness, numbness and bewilderment. The grief was tangible. No one had to speak. It affected how people walked and looked. As one executive said: 'It is as though someone has died!'

The grief of individuals and cultures can be expressed in various ways.

○ *Anticipated* grief occurs when people fear the loss that is to come. When I spoke to staff in one hospital, which had already drastically reduced staff numbers, people expressed fear that they would be next in line for redundancy. They dreaded trying to find alternative employment, being able to cover mortgages, pay school fees and health insurance. Some worried that, if they stayed, they would be assigned to different roles away from their friends; others feared that they were too old to learn new skills in the proposed restructured system.

○ *Cumulative grief overload* occurs when loss is experienced simultaneously from many sources. I believe that this is a particularly common experience for executives, managers and clinicians in healthcare systems in view of the constant changes imposed on them from above. In one hospital, for example, there had been many small changes and apparently everyone appeared to be coping. One day, however, the daily roster for resident doctors had to be slightly changed. Suddenly, to the surprise of the manager, there was an immediate, irrational outburst by several doctors. Angrily one doctor protested: 'We have had enough of all these…changes! No more! No more!' The roster alteration, small though it was, became the 'final straw'. When clinicians are under significant work pressure, such a reaction is in many ways understandable.

○ *Suppressed* grief happens when people and cultures are not encouraged to express their feelings of loss. Caregivers such as nurses and medical clinicians are constantly required to relate to suffering patients, their friends and relatives, but they are not permitted to express how they themselves feel.

○ *Chronic* or *fatalistic* grief takes place when people feel that nothing can be done or no one will listen to their feelings about their experience of loss. Cynicism and deep anger lurk beneath the surface. I believe that chronic grief plagues many healthcare systems today.

All these types of grief, if not understood and appropriately responded to, undermine morale and are bound to impact upon the welfare and safety of patients.

Guideline 7: During the process of merging organizations rituals of mourning are necessary to allow cultures and individuals to express their grief and move on

Give sorrow words: the grief that does not speak
Whispers the o'er-fraught heart, and bids it break.

(William Shakespeare)[28]

As explained in Chapter 1, we cannot live or communicate without rituals. Of particular concern here are what are called 'rites of passage', that is, rituals that not only *mark* the passing of one stage of life and entry into another, such as birth, marriage, death, but also *effect* the transition. For example, there is no way to become prime minister or a judge without a rite of induction. Of course, in an emergency a person can temporarily assume these roles, but at some point in order to be 'really in office' they will need a formal public ritual that leads them from a former status into their new role. The more important and threatening the transition the more formal will be the ritual. Rituals of mourning are rites of passage or processes in which loss and denial in the face of death are formally acknowledged, and the future

28   William Shakespeare, *Macbeth*, act IV, scene iii, p.209.

confronted with all its uncertainties, fears and hopes. John Bowlby considered rituals of mourning are positive if there is a successful effort by individuals 'to accept both that a change has occurred in the external world and that [they are] required to make corresponding changes in [their] internal representational world and to reorganize, and perhaps to reorient, [their] attachment behavior accordingly'.[29] The same can be said of any culture or organization that experiences grief. However, these rituals are not popular in Western cultures. Anthropologist Geoffrey Gorer concluded that rituals of loss are turned into rituals of denial. Grieving 'is treated as if it were a weakness, a self-indulgence, a reprehensible bad habit instead of a psychological necessity'.[30] Anything that is thought to express morbidity or death is anathema.[31] Gorer described this denial of loss as the 'pornography' of death, that is, noteworthy loss is not to be referred to in public; death and mourning are to be dealt with in private. So we are encouraged to use euphemisms when describing a person who has just died, for example, 'the person has passed away'.

This denial of loss has become an art form that is evident in contemporary industry, including healthcare institutions. William Lutz invented the term 'doublespeak' to describe ways in which language can be used in industry to hide the pain of loss. Euphemisms abound. People who lose their jobs are 'retrenched', 'dehired' or 'selected out' by firms that are 'downsizing', having 'workforce adjustments or restructuring'. In hospitals, patients can be encouraged to experience 'discomfort' rather than 'feeling pain'.[32] Of course, in healthcare facilities which are primarily concerned with healing people who are sick, the realities of dying and death can be indications of institutional breakdown. Hence, loss of any kind sits uncomfortably in the cultures of these institutions.[33] Little wonder if managers are ill equipped to cope with organizational losses. Yet to deny loss is to be haunted by it; as the Roman poet Ovid wrote: 'Suppressed grief suffocates.'[34] Readers may recall the phenomenal outpouring of grief at the time of Princess Diana's death. When she

29   John Bowlby (1980) *Loss: Sadness and Depression*. New York: Basic Books, p.18.
30   Geoffrey Gorer (1965) *Death, Grief and Mourning*. London: Crescent Press, p.85.
31   See Jessica Mitford (1963) *The American Way of Death*. New York: Simon & Schuster, pp.18–19.
32   See William Lutz (1987) *Doublespeak*. New York: Harper & Row, pp.1–21.
33   See Arbuckle 2000, p.318.
34   Ovid, *Tristia,* book V, eleg. 1, line 63.

died, there was a remarkable decrease in the number of people asking for help to overcome their depression. Psychiatrists concluded that the unparalleled public grieving permitted people to release deeply hidden emotions about some of their own personal issues.[35]

The following case study illustrates this intimate relationship between cultural and individual mourning. As long as cultural mourning is forbidden individuals must suppress their own feelings of loss. The public embrace of loss allows individual pain to be acknowledged and let go. Then new life is able to emerge.

CASE STUDY: CULTURAL AND INDIVIDUAL MOURNING

For many years there was an official and public refusal in the United States to admit the tragic mistakes and failure of the Vietnam war, as well as the bravery and suffering of thousands of soldiers. One summer I stumbled on this poorly written statement publicly displayed in the centre of a small New England village: 'Please understand that we are not asking for a parade, a monument or pity. But we do ask you to remember in your own way the 58,129 Americans who died in the war in Vietnam... We as individuals and as a nation learned something of human value for having been in SE Asia. The sacrifice we maintain was not futile.'

This is a poignant plea for the right to mourn publicly, the right to grieve and to learn from the lessons of defeat. The building of the national memorial in Washington, DC to the fallen has provided a chance for people to mourn because it is a public recognition that tragedies have occurred. As one commentator wrote: 'We left...so many men and women...without a funeral to give focus to our grief...without the ritual of saying goodbye. The Wall changed that; it is about the dead, but [also] for the living. The Wall...let us say goodbye.'[36]

---

35   Reported in *The Sydney Morning Herald* (17 December 1997), 12.
36   William Broyles (1986) 'A ritual for saying goodbye.' *US News and World Report* (10 November), 19.

Guideline 8: The rituals of mourning in the merging process, under appropriate leaders, will involve three stages: separation, liminality and reaggregation

Every merger will entail loss and this must be safely and positively 'managed' through rituals. The process of merging cultures constitutes a rite of passage or ritual of initiation in which participants are invited to move beyond the contradictory impulses that loss evokes in order to embrace a new cultural identity. On the one hand, the cultures to be merged feel the urge to cling tenaciously to what is lost and had given them meaning and a sense of identity. On the other hand, now they must build a new type of life and relationships. What was positive in the past is to be retained while the new is to be embraced. The ever present danger is to give way to the first impulse, with the result that the merger fails. John Keats described the ideal ritual of grieving, that is, the process of letting go the old and embracing the new (which he calls 'die into life') in this way:

> Most like the struggle at the gate of death
> Or liker still to one who should take leave
> Of pale, immortal death
> And with a pang as hot as death is chill
> With fierce convulse, die into life.[37]

Anthropologist Victor Turner, building on the earlier insights of Arnold Van Gennep, identified three cultural stages in the process of ritual initiation into a new identity: the separation from *societas*, through *liminality*, and finally *re-entry* to *societas*, but with a new and invigorating identity.

By *societas* he means a culture in which there is role differentiation, structure, segmentation and a hierarchical system of institutionalized positions. Most cultures, including healthcare, approximate to this type. The first stage of the ritual of initiation is the process of separation from *societas*; this is marked by a feeling of sadness, denial, fear of letting go the past. There can be a yearning or nostalgia for what has been or is about to be lost, a restlessness, despair and an anger that can be directed against organizational leaders or fellow workers. *Liminality*, on the other hand, is a type of culture which is undifferentiated,

---

37   John Keats (1899) 'Hyperion.' In *The Complete Poetical Works of Keats*, Book 3. Boston, MA: Houghton Mifflin, pp.211–212.

homogeneous, in which individuals meet each other integrally or as one human being to another, not segmented into status and roles. It is the phase of 'cultural nakedness', a cultural *tabula rasa*, sometimes referred to as the *chaos* or the *betwixt-and-between* stage, in which the cultures that must merge feel both attracted by the security of the past and the call to face the future. Former identities must be abandoned in order to embrace the new cultural identity. It is a self-reflexive stage, a search for, and ownership of, a new or common mythology that gives people a new identity and purpose. This is the particularly dangerous stage, when the risk of escaping back to the past or of becoming paralysed by the chaos is extremely great. *Re-entry* into the new *societas* constitutes the third stage of organizational grieving. The bereaved cultures are able to reflect on what has been lost with some degree of marked detachment. The new culture is slowly emerging; there is even a sense of excitement and energy as people look to the future.[38]

Traditional cultures: Lessons in rituals of grieving

The way in which a people's culture deals with physical bereavement sets the pattern for how people cope with significant losses. In traditional cultures people are especially aware of the fact that a community has a life of its own. When, for example, a death occurs, the entire community, not just particular individuals, is affected. A set of relationships is destroyed by the death, and a new set must be established if the community is to hold together and survive. If the death is unacknowledged, the new order or relationships cannot emerge. Emile Durkheim (1885–1917), a founding father of anthropology, wrote that 'Mourning is not a natural movement of private feelings wounded by a cruel loss; it is a duty imposed by the group.'[39] No member of a traditional culture is allowed to be indifferent to a death in their midst because it needs to be formally acknowledged that when one person dies, in a sense the entire group dies. Those who feel no personal sorrow will nonetheless be expected to weep, and even inflict suffering and inconvenience on themselves. By collectively mourning, the members express their belief that the group itself is suffering grief, and in doing so they overcome and

---

38 See Turner 1967, p.99, and (1969) *The Ritual Process: Structure and Anti-Structure.* New York: Aldine, p.103.

39 Emile Durkheim (1965) *The Rules of Sociological Method,* trans. S. Solovay and J. Mueller. New York: Free Press, p.31.

repair the loss that has occurred. Durkheim's comment may appear to be rather cynical in denying to the mourners spontaneity of feeling, which will often be real enough, but he is right about the need for the community itself ritually to mourn.

Traditional cultures, therefore, teach contemporary cultures several significant lessons:

- All change is felt as catastrophic even when it is rationally understood to be an advantage, 'since it threatens the established and familiar order and requires new attitudes and behaviour, changes in relationships, a move into a comparatively unknown future'.[40]

- Rituals formally articulate that loss affects not only a particular individual within a culture, but the culture itself and all who belong to it.

- Without these rituals that name the reality of loss and articulate what the culture should become by means of a new founding mythology and set of internal relationships, the group is in considerable danger of becoming trapped in or haunted by the past.

- Certain important places and buildings, not just individuals, have lives of their own; they contain 'good' and 'bad' memories of the past. So, like individuals, they also experience loss when changes are made. Hence, the 'spirits' of these buildings, so intimately connected with living people, must also be the object and subject of rituals of mourning.[41]

- Unarticulated grief is like a powder keg waiting to be ignited into all kinds of culture-destroying behaviour, and that cannot be tolerated, so the following guideline is inherent in rituals of mourning: 'Holding on kills, letting go heals.'

- Ritual leaders, by directing individuals and cultures through the stages of grieving, show that it is possible for anxiety to be mastered in constructive ways so that realistic order can again be achieved while due respect is being paid to the past.

40 Lyth 1989, p.34.
41 For an example see Anne Salmond (1975) *Hui: A Study of Maori Ceremonial Gatherings.* Wellington, NZ: A.H. & A.W. Reed, pp.40–41.

○ Ritual leaders need to be officially appointed for the task from the group.

As explained in Chapter 1, ritual is the stylized or repetitive symbolic use of bodily movement and gesture within a social context to express and articulate meaning. Occurring within a social context where there is potential or real tension/conflict in social relations, it is performed to resolve or hide such tension. Rituals in traditional cultures, by not hiding the reality of loss, seek to resolve the tensions and conflicts to allow new life to emerge. There are normally two levels of oppositional, disengagement/engagement processes at work within traditional mourning rituals. First, there is a ritual process that is directed at the deceased. The dead must be formally *disengaged* from the living; they are given permission, as it were, to leave this world and become *engaged* in relationships with other spirits elsewhere. They are assigned to a new, esteemed and safe status, that is tradition. Among the Australian Aboriginals and the Maori people in New Zealand, although the spirit is independent of flesh in a sense of outlasting their disunion, it is thought to haunt its former 'home'. It must be formally encouraged to 'move on' if it is to become an honoured ancestor in tradition. The second set of disengagement/engagement rituals relate directly to the living. They must formally become *disengaged* from the negative influences of the deceased and *engage* themselves in forming a new set of social relationships or culture.[42]

These two processes in traditional cultures take place within a span of the three stages already described: the separation stage in which rituals vigorously encourage the community to admit that death has occurred; the liminality stage in which the community especially concentrates over a lengthy period of time on the two processes of disengagement and engagement. Finally, rituals mark the end of mourning and the community must now concentrate on living out the new set of social relationships.[43]

In summary, traditional rites of passage respond to the needs of the bereaved at three levels: the psychological, mythological and

42 See Kenneth Maddock (1974) *The Australian Aborigine: A Portrait of their Society.* Harmondsworth: Penguin, pp.158–176, and Salmond 1975, pp.179–194.
43 See helpful insights by David M. Noer (1993) *Healing the Wounds: Overcoming the Trauma of Layoffs and Revitalizing Downsized Organizations.* San Francisco, CA: Jossey-Bass, pp.130–133; Jean Hartley and John Benington (2010) *Leadership for Healthcare.* Bristol: Policy Press, pp.61–73; and William Bridges (1995) *Jobshift.* London: Nicholas Brealey Publishing, pp.120–123.

sociological. At the psychological level, people require a ritual that culturally permits or encourages them to express fully and openly their feelings of loss. The public sharing of loss is one critically important way for the reality of loss to be accepted. People need also to see meaning in their loss, so in the ritual cultural myths are articulated that both console and challenge the bereaved to reflect on the future. At the sociological level, the bereaved need to feel that their grief is understood and shared by others, and that, at the right moment, they can return to society with new life and be fully accepted by it. We in the Western world can well learn about the importance of ritual from people of traditional cultures.

EXAMPLE: TRADITIONAL MOURNING RITUAL

In New Zealand, a new hospital had been built to replace an older, smaller and less-equipped one some miles away. While the new hospital had undoubtedly superior medical services, nonetheless people had long attachments to the old hospital and had strong negative feelings about abandoning it. The local Maori people, many of whom had been patients and/ or workers at the old hospital, were invited to lead the ritual of opening of the new hospital following the rather brief and austere welcoming speech of the local member of parliament. By contrast the Maori ritual lasted two days; the first day's ritual was held at the old hospital with particular emphasis being given to the disengagement of the spirits of the old hospital and their engagement in the world of tradition. The ritual language was direct and unambiguous: 'Go to your ancestors!' This was not disrespectful to the spirits of the old hospital; on the contrary, it was a recognition that the spirits had the right to leave the living and go to join the noble state of the ancestors and stop any haunting of the living. In between the ritual speeches people spontaneously told stories of their experiences of the hospital, a place where they had been born, relatives had died and friends been healed. On the second day, the crowd moved to the site of the new hospital. While the spirits of the old hospital continued to be encouraged to leave, the emphasis, however, was on welcoming the new spirits to

---

> the hospital alongside the process of taking ownership of the
> new hospital. This became a joyous experience, with people
> reflecting on the positive advantages of the newly opened
> hospital. The day ended with a large banquet for all present.

Application to healthcare mergers

Chief executive team members and/or their officially appointed and
trained delegates are to be the ritual leaders of the rites of passage
whereby the cultures to be merged become one encompassing
organizational culture. In a true sense, team members are not the
doers of ritual but are *themselves* the ritual. That is, by the example of
their acceptance of the new founding mythology of the merging
organization, they are to make a reality of the idea that another way of
being and acting *is* possible. Myth specialist Joseph Campbell described
the ritual leader of cultural change in this way: he or she is a 'hero',
who 'ventures forth from the world of common day into a region of...
wonder: fabulous forces are encountered and a decisive victory is won.
The hero comes back from this mysterious adventure with the power to
bestow boons on his fellow man [*sic*].'[44] The ritual leader is a hero who
has visited, and been converted to the mythology and values of a new
culture; their behaviour will mirror this interior transformation. Hence
the task of executive team members is to prove by their behaviour
that the destination of the merging culture can be reached. Other staff
members will recognize that the executive team members are carrying
within themselves the vision of the ultimate merger, and are drawn
to follow them with confidence. If the conversion of executive team
members to the new founding mythology and vision proves to be
mere rhetoric, and if the team members are not prepared to lead the
rites of passage to a new organizational culture, people will quickly
become cynical. The merging process is then put at grave risk.

---

44   Joseph Campbell (1949) *The Hero with a Thousand Faces.* Princeton, NJ: Princeton University
     Press, p.30.

TABLE 6.1: CULTURAL GRIEVING IN MERGERS

Merger: Ritual stages of cultural initiation	Executive leaders: Cultural ritual leaders
Stage 1: Separation from *societas* culture:	**Founding communications:**
Initial shock and reactions, e.g. sadness, fear of letting go the past, denial, nostalgia, anger, resistance	Chief executive team clarifies, internalizes and models by actions new common mythology: vision/mission/values Formal public rituals to announce merger Communicates *clearly* and often: • acknowledging people's shock and fears • provides new mythology/values to staff merger timetable • is readily available to patiently listen to grief of staff • clarifies roles/training programmes for managers • provides prompt and just compensation for any displaced staff, plus counselling for new employment • pays particular attention to the needs of the less powerful groups affected
Stage 2: Liminality culture:	**Encouraging communications:**
Critical and lengthy state Decision: either escape to the past, or be paralysed by chaos of uncertainties, risk the new Process of disengaging from the past and engaging with the common founding mythology/values of the new culture: storytelling dynamic	• continues previous communications • establishes small groups to discuss through storytelling process new common mythology/values and implications for behaviour • schedules public rituals to mark stages of merger • seeks staff involvement in rituals
Stage 3: Re-entry to *societas*:	**Celebratory communications:**
Bereaved cultures: growing detachment from past cultural identities Interiorization of new common mythology/values *slowly* developing	• continues previous communications • celebratory rituals to mark achievements always connecting them to new mythology • publicizes emerging culture examples of team ownership of new mythology

What should the rituals of mourning or rites of passage contain? Table 6.1 describes the three stages of these rituals, namely separation, liminality and re-entry, and the way the official cultural ritual guides need to adapt their communications according to the requirements of each ritual stage. In stage 1, once the chief executive team has clarified and internalized the mythology of the new culture, formal communications to the cultures to be merged begin. They will include: the decision and reasons for the merger; an acknowledgement that this will cause staff members anxieties about their future; clarification of new roles; and an assurance people will be justly compensated for any redundancies, with particular attention being given to the needs of the less powerful groups that might be affected. Listening and communication can never be overdone in the merging process, as the anxieties of people may make it difficult for them to hear what is being said. Then comes the most lengthy and critical stage, the experience of liminality, the betwixt-and-between phase. Staff of both cultures are encouraged to disengage from the past and engage with the new. This process of developing a new cultural identity through storytelling (see Chapter 1, Guideline 10) cannot be rushed and it demands very sensitive ritual leadership. Ample space must be given to people to tell their stories of the past and express their hopes for the future. Do people see positive signs of a new culture beginning to emerge, however faintly? In the re-entry stage, ritual leaders need to concentrate on identifying and celebrating positive signs of the new culture that are emerging.

CASE STUDY: GRIEVING RITUAL

I was once invited by the CEO of a large public hospital in Australia, after the government had decided to merge it with another hospital some distance away, to assist her with the process. I was officially delegated by her to meet with groups and individuals anywhere to listen to their fears and anxieties over the planned merger. At the same time, I constantly communicated to the hospital staff progress reports of the merger and the implications for employment. In her communications, she sympathetically acknowledged the fears that the merger evoked; she assured staff that, if there were to be redundancies, the hospital would endeavour to find alternative employment opportunities. My involvement in the process lasted weeks. I made myself available to listen to people at times and places convenient to them. The two questions I asked were: What do you feel about the forthcoming merger? and Do you see any positive qualities to the proposed merger? During the first weeks, the first question was dominant, but as time elapsed people were prepared to grapple with the second. During the process, staff members frequently expressed gratitude for the willingness of the CEO and other executives to give them the space to express their feelings and, at the same time, to continue communicating to them the reality of the challenges and progress of the merger. It was a process that respected people's dignity and testified to the authenticity of the hospital's commitment to care for their staff.

Guideline 9: Considerable time and effort must be directed at helping managers to develop their new roles as culture change-agents

This guideline applies equally to senior and middle management and clinical roles. Managers have a vested interest in maintaining the status quo; they achieved their status and power through acquiring and exercising particular skills and behaviours under the old organizational cultures. Nothing will happen if they are not committed to cultural change and have, or are not taught, the skills to lead the merging process.[45]

Summary

- The term 'merger' is commonly loosely used to cover such organizational changes as joint ventures, strategic alliances, networks, horizontal or vertical acquisitions, partnerships and restructuring. It refers to the process whereby organizations dialogue as equals, with the intention of producing a single new entity with its own culture, not infrequently with a new name. Whether the term is used loosely or strictly, however, some degree of cultural change is required.

- Despite the popularity of mergers, it is rare that they ever achieve their desired potential. When mergers succeed or fail,

---

45   See Oram and Wellins 1995, p.129.

cultural issues should always be examined for an explanation. It is easy to plan and introduce structural changes to support mergers, but they will not be effective if the cultural issues are not addressed. Mergers require mythological changes that affect a people's feelings and identities, but it needs to be recognized that such changes are slow and uncertain.

○ In every successful merger, a new culture develops with its own mythological support base. This means that cultures that seek to merge must be prepared to give up cherished elements of their existing identity. It is virtually impossible for leaders to over-communicate in a merger process, simply because people are able to let go and adjust to change more easily if they are able to face the known rather than the unknown. Communications must be honest, and apologies must be made if incorrect information has been given.[46]

○ In any merger process, individuals and cultures can experience grief, flowing from loss. Unless the grief of cultures is addressed individuals are unable to deal publicly with their own feelings of loss. Unarticulated grief will obstruct the process of merging organizational cultures. Cultural mourning involves a ritual of initiation, that is, disengagement from the past and engagement with a new, energizing mythology.

○ There are traditionally three stages to the mourning process: separation, liminality and re-entry. The leaders of this journey must respond appropriately to each phase. The second and most critical stage is liminality, that is, the letting go of the old and the development of openness to the new. Integral to this stage is allowing people to express their feelings of loss, their anxieties and hopes for the future.

Strategic implications

Policies

○ Mergers and any form of restructuring, no matter how objectively important, normally evoke all kinds of anxieties

---

46   See comments by Wall and Wall 2000, pp.177–190.

among employees. It is essential that senior executives and managers formulate policies to guide the merging process according to the foundational values of healthcare such as justice and compassion.

○ Employees need to be kept fully informed of the process and its implications for their welfare. At the same time, as people and cultures can feel a deep sense of loss as a consequence of mergers, policies to guide the merging process must include rituals of organizational and individual grieving.

Implementation

○ While communication at all stages of a merger is the key to its success, senior executives will realize that nothing can substitute for willingness to communicate personally with employees rather than relying only on impersonal memos or handouts. Communications by outside consultants are no substitute for the personal involvement of senior executives.

○ This means that senior executives must first be convinced of the reasons for the merger and then be prepared to listen to and dialogue with employees about their concerns; what will most worry employees will be issues such as their security of employment. The more executives are prepared to listen and enter into real dialogue with employees the more people will accept ownership of the cultural changes. Failure by senior executives to be transparent will only increase the general anxiety of employees and further undermine their trust in executives.

○ Culturally sensitive senior executives and managers will be aware that not just individuals but the organizational culture itself will experience the symptoms of grief. This means that formal and informal grieving processes, under the direction of skilled leaders, will need to be established throughout the stages of the merger.

CHAPTER 7

Faith-Based Healthcare

Case Study

> Business people often think nonprofit organizations spend too much time agonizing about their mission. But in fact it's time well spent, because that's how a nonprofit builds a sense of community and shared values.
>
> (F. Warren McFarlan)[1]

> [Non-profit institutions] exist for the sake of their mission, and this must never be forgotten.
>
> (Peter Drucker)[2]

This chapter explains:

- the meaning and purpose of faith-based healthcare organizations
- that 'the mission' is to be the driving force in all decision-making
- that the identity of faith-based healthcare is threatened by the demands of big business as well as by changing values in society
- that, in partnering with governments there are positive benefits, but also significant risks
- that faith-based organizations must be proactive in selecting and forming staff according to their founding story and values.

---

1   F. Warren McFarlan (1999) 'Working on nonprofit boards: Don't assume the shoe fits.' *Harvard Business Review* 77, 6, 77.

2   Peter Drucker (1990) *Managing the Nonprofit Organization: Practices and Principles.* New York: HarperCollins, p.45.

Faith-based organizations are significantly religious in nature and generally non-profit, as compared to commercial, government or private secular institutions. Like other non-profits, they are self-governing, attracting a substantial amount of voluntary contributions, while serving public purposes as well as meeting the common goals of the people involved. For centuries, since the second century AD, Christian healthcare hospitals and allied facilities have flourished in the Western world, with particular emphasis on the needs of people who are socially and economically poor.[3] In the United States, the proportion of hospitals that remain non-profit is well over 80 per cent, with the vast majority sponsored by religious denominations. In countries like Britain, where there is publicly funded healthcare, the great majority of hospitals are government owned but, given the rising costs of healthcare, governments are anxious to encourage the development of non-profit and faith-based hospitals. This chapter examines faith-based healthcare institutions, their successes and the increasing challenges they face in maintaining their primary emphasis on their mission.

This analysis of faith-based healthcare institutions will focus on facilities sponsored by the Roman Catholic Church in the United States, Canada and Australia. The insights and conclusions, however, are generally relevant to all faith-based initiatives. Since we are dealing with faith-based institutions, it will be necessary at times to explain briefly some of the theological issues that have to be taken into account if these institutions contract with governments or for-profit agencies to provide healthcare services.

Provision of healthcare services by the Catholic Church

The investment by the Catholic Church in healthcare services is staggering. In Australia, Catholic services form the largest non-government source of health and aged care services, including 75 hospitals, of which 21 are public hospitals directly financed by

---

3   For example, see Geoff Foster (2010) *Study of the Response by Faith-Based Organizations to Orphans and Vulnerable Children – Preliminary Summary Report*, UNICEF. Accessed 18 June 2012 at www.jlica.org/pdf/unicefwrcpstudy.pdf; Amanda Porterfield (2005) *Healing in the History of Christianity*. Oxford: Oxford University Press, pp.43–91, and Ferngren 2009, pp.64–152.

state governments, several world-class research institutes, and 550 government-aided residential and community aged care services. In Canada the Catholic Church owns and manages 87 public hospitals. In the United States, the Catholic Church owns 11 per cent of the hospitals, provides 16 per cent of all community hospital admissions, and employs approximately 800,000 workers. By acute care bed count, 3 of the 10 largest healthcare systems in the United States are Catholic, as are 7 of the 10 largest non-profit systems. In addition there are 1796 continuing nursing facilities, home care and hospice care services. Though many of these services are heavily dependent on Medicare and Medicaid financing, Catholic and other voluntary hospitals have been 'bearing the brunt of caring for the uninsured population'.[4]

According to their mission statements Catholic healthcare services publicly commit themselves to live the values of the founding story of healthcare, namely the Good Samaritan parable. For example, in Sydney, Australia St Vincent's and Mater Health espouse the following core values: compassion, justice, human dignity, excellence, unity, mercy, hospitality and respect, while St John of God Health, which includes 14 hospitals, commits to: hospitality, compassion, respect, justice and excellence. In the United States, Catholic Health East, which includes 33 acute care hospitals, lists its core values as: reverence for each person, community, justice, commitment to those who are poor, courage, integrity; Catholic Health Initiatives: compassion, reverence, integrity and excellence.

According to available research, patients feel these values are being lived. For example, in New South Wales, Australia, the Catholic Church owns and manages two high-profile public hospitals for the state government; in 2010 both facilities ranked as two of the top eight hospitals in the state for patient satisfaction.[5] In 2010 a Thomson Reuters study of 225 health systems in the United States showed that 'Catholic and other church-owned systems are significantly more likely to provide higher quality performance and efficiency...than investor-owned systems.' As regards specifically Catholic health systems, it was found that they are 'significantly

---

4   See Barbra M. Wall (2011) *American Catholic Hospitals: A Century of Changing Markets and Missions.* New Brunswick, NJ: Rutgers University Press, p.118.

5   See Bureau of Health Information (2010) *Insights into Care: Patients' Perspectives on NSW Public Hospitals.* Sydney: NSW Government, p.19.

more likely to provide higher quality performance...than secular not-for-profit health systems'.[6] The research implies that facilities owned by churches may be the most active in ensuring their mission actively influences their decision-making throughout their systems. Earlier research in the United States concluded that the non-profit systems commonly provide services at lower cost, higher quality, and with greater efficiency, when compared with the for-profit services.[7]

Despite this positive evaluation, faith-based healthcare institutions have an uncertain future, with Catholic facilities particularly facing additional challenges. Cultural, economic and political forces, in addition to internal problems, increasingly threaten their ability to maintain the primary emphasis on the mission as the driving force in all decision-making.[8] They, like other non-profit institutions, are in constant danger of 'forgetting that the most important measure of success is the achievement of mission-related objectives, not [their] financial wealth or stability'.[9]

The history of faith-based educational institutions is not encouraging. The faith-based quality of educational establishments like Oxford, Cambridge, Harvard, Yale and Princeton has long since disappeared. In fact, at times these institutions have been openly hostile towards their Christian roots.[10] Even contemporary Catholic universities and colleges in the United States and elsewhere are in danger of experiencing the same fate.[11] Some in the United States believe the volume, momentum and complexity of change in healthcare is accelerating at such an alarming rate that it is becoming impossible

---

6   See David Foster (2010) *Research Brief: Differences in Health System Quality Performance by Ownership.* Thomson Reuters, 9 August. Accessed on 10 August 2010 at www.100tophospitals. com/assets/100TOPSystemOwnership.pdf, p.1.

7   See Stephen Duckett (2001) 'Does it matter who owns health facilities?' *Journal of Health Services Research and Policy 6,* 1, 59–62; Richard Lewis, Peter Hunt and David Carson (2006) *Social Enterprise and Community-Based Care.* London: King's Fund, p.10.

8   See Arbuckle 2000, pp.xi–xxiii; Leonard J. Nelson (2009) *Diagnosis Critical: The Urgent Threats Confronting Catholic Health Care.* Huntington, IN: Our Sunday Visitor, pp.9–22, 79–130.

9   J. Gregory Dees (1999) 'Enterprising Nonprofits.' In *Harvard Business Review on Nonprofits.* Boston, MA: Harvard Business School Publishing, p.164.

10   See George Marsden (1994) *The Soul of the American Academy: From Protestant Establishment to Established Nonbelief.* New York: Oxford University Press; George M. Marsden and Bradley J. Longfield (eds) (1992) *The Secularization of the Academy.* New York: Oxford University Press.

11   See James T. Burtchaell (1998) *The Dying of the Light: The Disengagement of Colleges and Universities from their Christian Churches.* Grand Rapids, MN: William B. Eerdmans, pp.557–742; Philip Gleason (1995) *Contending with Modernity: Catholic Higher Education in the Twentieth Century.* New York: Oxford University Press; Melanie M. Morey and John J. Piderit (2005) *Catholic Higher Education: A Culture in Crisis.* Oxford: Oxford University Press.

for faith-based healthcare to be true to its founding mission and values. Jesuit Richard McCormack, a well-respected Notre Dame University theologian, shocked supporters of Catholic hospitals in 1995 when he stated 'the mission has become impossible'.[12] The reasons he gave have not disappeared. Indeed they have intensified. It is well worth exploring the reasons for concern in the following section.

Reasons for concern

1. 'Corrupted' values

Given the pressures that faith-based institutions are facing it is relatively easy for them to accept uncritically the values of the marketplace. When this happens, concluded McCormack, 'any sense of mission can be smothered by bottom-line thinking'. The ability to 'treat the indigent will disappear'.[13] The majority of hospitals have resisted the pressures to capitulate to market values, but the temptation to do so remains ever present.

2. Financial challenges

Market forces are making it increasingly difficult for hospitals in general, especially in poor rural and city centres of the United States, to remain financially viable. With consumers, employers, government and commercial players increasing their demands for lower costs, higher quality, better access and more information about outcomes, most hospitals over the last 20 years have taken a series of competitive initiatives to retain and, if possible, improve their market positions. Between 1980 and 2009 approximately 2000 hospitals closed. In the period 1990 to 2009 the number of hospital emergency departments declined by 27 per cent.[14] As facilities under financial pressures reduce their services or close, the remaining hospitals are swamped, particularly with uninsured patients.

It is not surprising, therefore, that faith-based healthcare institutions are also feeling the pressure. In 2001 the British publication

---

12 Richard A. McCormick (1995) 'The Catholic hospital today: Mission impossible.' *Origins 25*, 20, 649.
13 Richard A. McCormick (1998) 'The end of Catholic hospitals.' *America* (4 July), 6, 8.
14 See Mary Brophy (2011) 'Study: ERs shrink as demand rises.' *USA Today* (17 May), 8.

The Economist claimed that 'It would not be surprising, a decade from now, if all non-profit hospitals (in the United States), except those with generous patrons or unusually competent managers, were closed or sold.'[15] The prophecy is being proved accurate. For example, the prestigious six-hospital Catholic Caritas Christi Health Care, Boston, was sold in 2011 for financial reasons to a New York-based private-equity firm for $US830 million. The iconic St Vincent's Hospital, Manhattan, closed in 2010. Those that continue commonly find it increasingly difficult to finance services for the poor. If they cease to provide this aid they cease to be true to their mission and lose their tax-exempt status; closure is the only option. In 2007 a large system, Catholic Health Care West, was forced to settle a lawsuit for $US473 million because uninsured patients complained that 'its hospitals were overcharging them and using aggressive debt collection techniques against them'.[16] Faith-based healthcare institutions risk adopting the values of their for-profit competitors in the pressure to survive.

3. Depersonalization

Faith-based hospitals have long prided themselves on their personalized services, that is, the willingness of clinicians and staff members to spend time with patients out of concern for holistic healing, which is increasingly, however, difficult to provide for technological and financial reasons. Technological improvements have substantially lessened the time patients stay in hospitals, so there is less time for personalized services to patients. For example, in the 1940s patients entering a hospital for myocardial infarction remained there for five to seven weeks, but today they stay for only a few days. More patients will be treated on a day only basis with an emphasis on efficient and rapid 'throughout' of patients through the system. Acute care hospitals are a diminishing focus of healthcare. Further, managed care, with its emphasis on keeping costs down, threatens to ignore the needs of ailing individuals to be listened to; clinicians must hurry to the next patient.

---

15 'Non-profits under pressure.' (2001) *The Economist* (27 January), 71.
16 Nelson 2009, p.203.

4. The risks of mergers

To survive financially, many hospitals in the United States engage in mergers and consolidations to achieve economies of scale and to better position themselves to negotiate with managed care organizations and other players. Traditionally, rival Catholic hospitals have moved to form centralized mega-systems with surprising speed over the last 20 years. While this solution may solve financial problems, it carries potential dangers. One of the strengths of faith-based hospitals in the past has been their links with local communities. People felt closely attached to these hospitals, and so often donated money and/or volunteered labour to support their mission. But the more mergers occur the more centralized their organizations become. In these circumstances personal connections with local communities weaken or disappear. Excessive centralization neuters local community involvement and ownership.

In the United States, for example, the 59 Catholic healthcare systems as a whole have now formed the largest non-government non-profit healthcare system in the nation.[17] But, as one American commentator wrote: 'In many cases, distinctiveness [of Catholic healthcare] is blurred. Even if [traditional] values…are driving institutions from within, those values are obscured by the public face of megasystems that rival the largest US for-profit corporations in financial scale.'[18] The front page of *The Wall Street Journal* in 1998 declared with obvious amazement that the Sisters of Charity National Health System, which owns some 40 hospitals, had reserves of $US2 billion in cash and investments. The article stated that it was 'one of the largest reserves of any non-profit hospital system in the country'.[19] The article failed to point out that the system was freely providing considerable assistance to poor patients.

---

17   See Arthur Jones (1995) 'Huge nonprofit system feels pressure to cut costs, merge or get bigger.' *National Catholic Reporter* (16 June), 12.

18   'Catholic health care poised between mission and money.' (1998) *National Catholic Reporter* Editorial (23 January), 36.

19   Monica Langley (1998) 'Nuns' zeal for profits shapes hospital chain, wins Wall Street fans.' *Wall Street Journal* (7 January), 1A.

5. Tribalism

While mergers continue among Catholic healthcare services, there is also an intensification of tribalism between traditional rivals. Catholic facilities compete with each other in order to survive. The Catholic Archdiocese of New York in the early 1990s undertook a feasibility study to investigate whether the majority of their health providers could unite into one single delivery network for the best advantage of patients. They were unwilling to do so. The pattern continues. An observer described the problem: 'I think the basic destabilizing truth...is that Catholic sponsors don't trust one another [to unite], and that sentiment also finds expression among the managements and medical staffs of our institutions and agencies.'[20]

6. Ethical conflicts

Faith-based hospitals, especially Catholic, are running into an increasingly antagonistic public health establishment with very different ethical values. Governments demand authority to impose conditions when they provide grants for projects. But, for example, a mandatory requirement for Catholic hospitals to provide abortion services could lead to their closure.[21] In late January 2012 this became a real possibility for the hundreds of hospitals and other institutions sponsored by the Catholic Church in the United States. The US Department of Health and Human Services decreed that the much-needed Patient Protection and Affordable Act of 2010 (see Chapter 2) would require all employers to provide preventative medical insurance services for women, including contraception, to their employees. Included in the contraception requirement would be contraceptives that could cause abortions and sterilizations. The mandate allowed for a small exemption for religious institutions, if they employed members of their own denomination and their services were primarily for followers of their own faith. The exemption did not include the innumerable hospitals, welfare facilities, universities and other educational institutions that serve and employ vast numbers of people who are not Catholic. Protests against the mandate were immediate and vigorous. Influential Catholic groups claimed that the

20   Patricia Cahill (1994) 'Collaboration among Catholic health providers.' *Origins 24*, 12, 213.
21   See Nelson 2009, pp.151–162; Wall 2011, pp.103–126, 155–174.

decree violated their beliefs and they would have to withdraw from all involvement in healthcare and education. The decree also evoked widespread political uproar among people who are not Catholic, claiming that it violated the principles of religious liberty. Within two weeks President Obama had softened the decree; religiously affiliated educational institutions and hospitals would not be forced to offer contraception coverage to their employees. Instead, insurers would be required to offer full free coverage to any women who work in such institutions.[22]

7. Storytellers

Traditionally, Catholic healthcare institutions were mainly staffed by unpaid members of religious orders. Formed and trained for the task, these people were the highly visible carriers of the founding story of healthcare. This is no longer the case as their numbers have so radically declined that it is increasingly rare to find representatives of these orders in a hospital, even at the level of trustees. In 1959, for example, one Catholic hospital in Australia was staffed almost entirely by 259 religious nuns. Today, there are no nuns on the staff. Religious orders do not have the numbers, nor will they have them ever again. They may still *own* hospitals, but their involvement is increasingly being reduced to that of remote trustees and even this role is rapidly passing into lay hands.[23] Consequently, there is no longer any guarantee that staff members, even at the highest executive levels, are members of the Catholic Church or indeed, have any commitment to its founding values of healthcare.

8. Governing boards

A governing board is 'an organized group of people with the authority collectively to control and foster an institution that is usually administered by a qualified executive and staff'.[24] That is, the task of boards is to formulate policies in view of their vision,

---

22   See 'Obama's "war on religion".' (2012) *The Economist* (11 February), 40; 'Obama adjusts a rule covering contraceptives.' (2012) *Times Digest* (11 February), 1.

23   See Arbuckle 2000, pp.222–239; Nelson 2009, pp.85–89.

24   Cyril O. Houle (1997) *Governing Boards: Their Nature and Nuture*. San Francisco, CA: Jossey-Bass, p.6.

mission, and values and consequently to call an institution to be accountable. However, governing boards of non-profit institutions do not have a good history. Observers once remarked that 'Effective governance by a board of a non-profit organization is a rare and unnatural action.'[25] In my experience there are many reasons for this: traditionally, members are selected not on the basis of skills and values, but because they represent groups of the communities that surround the healthcare institutions; poor formation of members in the vision, mission and values of the institutions; failure to clarify the role of the board; and neglecting to call CEOs to be accountable to the vision, mission and values of the organizations. For example, unless board members are watchful, it is easy for a CEO, not necessarily deliberately, to withhold information necessary for good decision-making.

9. Identity crisis

The mission of Catholic healthcare facilities is no longer as sharply defined, causing significant confusion for board members, CEOs and other executive staff. During the nineteenth century and until the mid-1960s, Catholics formed a minority group, subject to significant prejudice and discrimination. Consequently, educational and healthcare services were to be 'citadels and fortresses for the preservation of the faith in a hostile external environment characterized by a dominant Protestant order, continuing anti-Catholic prejudice and the growing influence of secularisation'.[26] For this reason, the Church's symbols of identity in all its many institutions remained relatively static, universal and sharply defined. Recall, for example, the unique religious habits of nuns, or the rule that Catholics should not eat meat on Fridays, that they should not worship with or marry members of other faiths and denominations, that liturgies were conducted in Latin. In the United States the Church had become so successful that it had become 'the best organized and most powerful of the nation's subcultures – a source of both

---

25   Barbara Taylor, Richard P. Chait and Thomas P. Holland (1996) 'The new work of the nonprofit board.' *Harvard Business Review* 74, 5, 36.

26   Gerald Grace (2002) *Catholic Schools: Mission, Markets and Morality.* London: RoutledgeFalmer, p.7. See also Christopher J. Kauffman (1995) *Ministry and Meaning: A Religious History of Catholic Health Care in the United States.* Chestnut Ridge, NY: Crossroads Publishing, p.138.

alienation and enrichment for those born within it and an object of bafflement or uneasiness for others'.[27] An average Catholic hospital was akin to a parish – with chapel, religious symbols, chaplains, daily religious services. There was no need for a mission statement because the purpose of the facilities was clear to all to see and experience. Not infrequently, however, unlike the schools, Catholic hospitals and other healthcare services were open to any person in need, no matter what their religion.[28] Free assistance to the poor was financially possible because special hospitals were provided for the wealthy who then subsidized the outreach services for the poor.

Since the mid-1960s, however, this clear-cut traditional Catholic identity of these hospitals has suddenly and radically changed. The rigid boundaries of the Church's identity collapsed under the combined impact of dramatic internal and external changes beginning in the 1960s: the remarkable achievements of Catholic education, the rise of welfare states, the theological and cultural impact of Vatican II (1963–5), the rapidly escalating costs of healthcare and the consequences of postmodernity. The Catholic educational system had become so successful that Catholics were able to move up into economic, social and political positions of power that had formerly been closed to them. By the early 1980s, for example, in the United States, the Irish had become the most financially successful of all non-Jewish ethnic groups.[29] The descendants of two centuries of immigrants ceased to be outsiders. Sociologically they had become 'indistinguishable as a group from their fellow citizens in terms of ethical values, social mores, and cultural tastes'.[30] At the same time, the rise of the welfare state led to universal healthcare in most Western countries, except in the United States. Thus, one primary reason for the establishment of Catholic healthcare services, namely to provide help for people who are poor, disappeared. In addition to these changes, the Vatican II Council theologically undermined the traditional symbols, mythology and rituals of post-Reformation Catholic identity. The new world of the Council was not to be

27   John Cogley (1974) *Catholic America*. New York: Image, p.135.

28   Local bishops did not always agree with this policy. For example, see Margaret M.K. O'Sullivan (1995) *A Cause of Trouble'? Irish Nuns and English Clerics*. Sydney: Crossing Press, p.225.

29   See John A. Coleman (1982) *An American Strategic Theology*. New York: Paulist, p.168.

30   Mark S. Massa (1999) *Catholics and American Culture*. New York: Crossroad, p.10.

considered inherently evil, Catholics must collaborate for a just world with people of goodwill everywhere, whether believers or not. Gone were the static identity markers.

These dramatic changes evoked significant disruption of identity for Catholics and their institutions; the fall-out continues to evoke identity crises for the Church's social and healthcare services.[31] The mission of Catholic healthcare facilities is no longer sharply defined. To add to the confusion, the changes of Vatican II happened to coincide with the dramatic upheaval of the cultural revolution of the 1960s in which every value and institution was subjected to questioning.[32] Catholic institutions and their staff members, already bewildered by internal changes to their Church, were now exposed to a secular world of mixed values and the rejection of modernity.

10. Government involvement

Governments, traditionally, tended to keep faith-based institutions at a distance, but since the 1980s there has generally been a significant reversal of this policy. Governments, when faced with the rising costs of social and healthcare services, are deliberately seeking the assistance of the non-profit sector. This new policy, referred to as 'faith-based initiatives',[33] is a partnership between governments and faith-based organizations whereby the latter provide social and healthcare services by accessing public moneys, while maintaining their religious identity. Governments seek the financial assistance of the voluntary sector; at the same time, they recognize that many non-profits have the expertise in leadership and management they desperately need.[34] It is assumed, however, that in collaborative projects, while faith-based groups are able to retain their specific

---

31 See Gerald A. Arbuckle (1993) *Refounding the Church; Dissent for Leadership.* Maryknoll, NY: Orbis, pp.43–66.

32 See Arbuckle 2004, pp.157–173.

33 See Arthur E. Farnsley (2007) 'Faith-Based Initiatives.' In James A. Beckford and N.J. Demerath (eds) *The Sage Handbook of the Sociology of Religion.* London: Sage Publications, pp.345–356. For example, the British Government established an Office of the Third Sector (OTS) in 2006 to support the environment for a thriving third sector, enabling the sector to campaign for change, cooperatives and public services, promote social enterprise and strengthen communities.

34 See 'Profiting from non-profits.' (2010) *The Economist* (17 July), 60.

religious character they cannot use government funding directly for religious purposes.

The former US president George W. Bush and former British Prime Minister Tony Blair proactively sought closer collaboration with faith-based institutions.[35] British Prime Minister David Cameron spoke of the Big Society.[36] He claimed that the state is too big, too intrusive. It should be smaller and smarter. To achieve this aim the state needs to utilize the power of intermediary institutions such as the family, schools, faith-based organizations and other voluntary agencies. Cameron and others often use the expression 'social entrepreneurship' to highlight a unique quality of faith-based and other non-profit organizations. A social entrepreneur identifies a social problem and engages entrepreneurial principles to invent, organize and manage a project to achieve social change. While a business entrepreneur assesses performance in terms of profit, a social entrepreneur emphasizes the creation of social capital.

CASE STUDY: BROMLEY BY BOW CENTRE

This facility was started by Andrew Mawson, a minister of the United Reformed Church, who was invited to a small and dilapidated church in East London. He opened up the area to the community and formed creative partnerships with local people and various organizations.[37] The centre has developed a distinctive method of developing and managing integrated community health services. It consists of a wide variety of statutory health services, community regeneration programmes, arts, education and social enterprise activity, with over 2000 people passing through weekly.[38]

Faith-based institutions can benefit from closer ties with governments, in addition to financial help. They must be financially and professionally accountable for their services, a requirement that

---

35 See Home Office (2004) *Working Together: Co-operation between Government and Faith Communities*. London: Home Office Faith Communities.
36 See Jesse Norman (2010) *The Big Society: The Anatomy of the New Politics*. Buckingham: University of Buckingham Press.
37 See Mawson 2008.
38 See Commission on Urban Life and Faith (2006) *Faithful Cities: A Call for Celebration, Vision and Justice*. Peterborough: Methodist Publishing House, p.70.

has not always been the case in the past. In the United States, the government, following the pattern set by many other governments, is insisting that faith-based hospitals now indicate the amount they spend on charity care and other community benefits, how much bad debt is really charity care and how they assess community needs. They are expected to demonstrate that they deserve the privileges of tax-exemption, government grants and charitable donations. In brief, higher levels of financial transparency are now required.[39] On the negative side, governments rarely understand the mission and values of faith-based groups.[40] Consequently there can be significant dangers for faith-based organizations, unless safeguards are in place, when they agree to collaborate with governments.

- They may lose their ability to critique governments' policies. Under the government of Prime Minister Howard in Australia (1996–2007), for example, only those non-profit (including faith-based) organizations that unquestionably accepted government policies continued to receive financial support for particular projects.[41]

- Partnering with faith-based institutions can be a way for governments to ignore their responsibilities that they alone should fulfil namely their obligations to develop an economy in which people have the right to employment, to healthcare and to welfare assistance when that is needed. When governments fail to accept this responsibility, they can blame voluntary agencies for their inability to take care of people in need. Experience shows that when an economy is faltering, the first groups to experience financial cutbacks will be these voluntary agencies. The poor suffer first and they have no political clout to protest.

---

39 See Julie Trocchio (2011) 'Get outside the tent: Embrace community.' *Health Progress 92*, 2, 33.
40 See comments by Davis *et al.* 2008, pp.50–56.
41 See Sarah Maddison, Richard Denniss and Clive Hamilton (2004) *Silencing Dissent: Non-Government Organisations and Australian Democracy*, Discussion Paper no. 65. Sydney: Australian Institute, pp.2–5.

⊙ Governments often expect success for immediate political advantage, but faith-based groups are conscious that radical cultural change demands a long-term commitment.

Options

In light of these pressures, Catholic healthcare institutions face an uncertain future regarding their identity and viability: Can the priority that needs to be given to the mission be reconciled with the realities of big business?[42] Can these institutions survive financially, if they wish to maintain a preferential concern for people who are poor, as their mission statements require? Can the founding story of Catholic healthcare, as articulated in the Good Samaritan parable, continue to inspire institutions now that the original carriers of the story are in rapid decline? In the mid-1990s, Jesuit moral theologian Richard McCormick contended that many non-profit hospitals in the United States, including Catholic facilities, would find it impossible to support themselves as competition for patients intensifies from for-profit facilities. He is increasingly being proved right.[43] He ended his prediction with this challenging question: 'How do we save the souls of these institutions as they manoeuvre through a competitive minefield?'[44]

These institutions have three options other than closing or selling to for-profit businesses. Option one is to re-state, unchanged, the symbols of their notably successful past. This nostalgic escape from reality is not a solution, as the qualities of Catholic identity must change as new situations emerge. History shows that the more rigid the defence of an untenable position, the more catastrophic the crash when it comes. Option two is to do nothing, that is, to go with the flow, uncritically accepting the values of the marketplace, abandoning all

---

42 See McCormick 1998, 5–11; Charles E. Curran (1997) 'The Catholic identity of Catholic institutions.' *Theological Studies 58*, 1, 90–108.

43 The Catholic Archdiocese of Boston is selling its Caritas Christi Health Care (the second largest health system in New England, comprising six hospitals) to a New York investment firm, Steward Healthcare System. According to the agreement 'their Catholic identities, and their existing policies on charitable and pastoral care, community benefits, and approach to labor relations form a social justice perspective' will be retained: 'Caritas Christi acquired by private investment firm.' *The Pilot* (Boston) (26/3/10). Accessed on 17 August 2010 at www.thebostonpolit.com/article.asp?ID=11605. On 30 April 2010, the 160-year old institution of St Vincent's Hospital in Manhattan, New York, closed after years of financial difficulties.

44 McCormick 1995, p.648.

uniqueness. According to this option, Catholic identity, it is argued, is too difficult to clarify and live by. Peter Steinfels, formerly religion editor of *The New York Times*, wrote that the real danger is that these healthcare institutions would mindlessly slip into an essentially secular, superficial image of their original religious identities, 'still bearing their insignia but no longer sharing the allegiance, their Catholic identity hollowed out and their links to...[their Catholic roots] reduced to historical memory and, maybe, the word "Saint" or "Catholic" at the portals'.[45] Significantly, a number of American Catholic hospitals today do not include Jesus Christ in their mission statements, on the assumption that his name alienates people.

Option three is to adopt the *refounding* process (see Chapter 5). In this option creative leaders are able to draw on their faith-based memories of the past but imaginatively express them in new symbols that are relevant to the present needs of people.[46] In the United States, for example, Catholic healthcare services will continue to emphasize advocacy for universal care.[47] In Australia and Britain the emphasis will be on improving access to good healthcare for marginalized people such as older people and those with disabilities, solo parents, indigenous people, asylum seekers. In brief, creative leaders will need to recognize and be personally committed to values that are identifiably Catholic.[48] They would need to be able to resolve the fundamental tension between the demands of the founding mission and values and financial viability in all healthcare.

But here is *the* problem. What does it mean to speak of 'values that are identifiably Catholic'? How are they to be explained and interiorized when the majority of staff members are either not Catholic or, if they nominally are, have little or no knowledge of, or interest in, the Catholic ethos? At the same time there can be no watering down of the radical demands of the Catholic understanding of holistic healing if the identity of their institutions is to remain clear. Steinfels commented that it does not seem acceptable to reduce Catholic identity to a few brief essentials, as in stating 'that Catholic hospitals abstain from performing abortions'. At the same time, he

45   Peter Steinfels (2003) *A People Adrift: The Crisis of the Roman Catholic Church in America.* New York: Simon & Schuster, p.114.
46   See Giddens 1992, p.75.
47   See US Bishops Conference (1993) 'Resolution on health reform.' *Origins 23*, 7, 98–102.
48   See John P. Beal (1994) 'Catholic hospitals: How Catholic will they be?' *Concilium 5*, 89.

wrote, it is not really 'satisfactory to recast that dimension in elevated but cloudy terms – respect, personal attention…so religiously neutral that they might easily apply to the Red Cross Blood Bank as to the Holy Cross Health Clinic'.[49] The radical qualities of compassion, equity, respect, justice, as understood by Catholic mythology, must be clearly defined and mirrored in the attitude and behaviour of staff members of healthcare institutions.

Practical guidelines

Given all the above, what would an anthropologist suggest to trustees, boards and executives of Catholic healthcare institutions and, by extension, to leaders of other faith-based healthcare services? The advice is summarized in a series of practical guidelines that I have found helpful when consulting to faith-based healthcare institutions. In this, I follow the advice of seventeenth-century philosopher René Descartes, who wrote that 'My design is not to teach the Method which everyone should follow in order to promote the good conduct of his reason, but only to show how I have endeavoured to conduct my own.'[50]

Guideline 1: Ensure that the mission drives decision-making

The fundamental tension in faith-based healthcare, as already explained, is between the mission and the business (see Chapter 2). Some may argue that business must take priority, that, without a margin, there can be no mission. The mission is then seen to be something secondary, even, at times, an obstacle to the achievement of good results in the business. When this occurs market economics or economic rationalism triumphs in decision-making. Others would claim that if we concentrate on the mission, the business will look after itself. Then the business is seen as something inferior to the mission. Both views are false and the polarization will lead to the

---

49   Steinfels 2003, pp.112–113.
50   René Descartes (1996) *Discourse on the Method and Meditations on First Philosophy*, ed. David Weissman, trans. Elizabeth Haldane and G.R. Ross. New Haven, CT: Yale University Press, p.4.

destruction of the uniqueness of Catholic and any other faith-based healthcare. The poles in the tension are complementary, but the mission is to be the senior partner, driving or permeating *all* decisions in the business side of facilities. The mission is not something to be considered from time to time; it must dynamically influence all activities. The mission is not to be limited to occasional rituals to mark the founder's day or to words in advertising literature or branding, but it must dynamically pervade the work and life of every section of a facility. There will always be a tension between the 'mission' and the 'business', but this can creatively be worked through in an atmosphere of dialogue.[51]

Carol Taylor, of Georgetown University, correctly argued that there must be no weakening of the specific Catholic identity in the mission statements of Catholic faith-based healthcare; nor should uniquely identifiable religious symbols and rituals be withdrawn. Unless mission statements are clearly Catholic, she insisted, it will not be possible in practice to sustain the specific emphasis on the mission and its inherent values. Language does matter in maintaining identity and in modelling behaviour.[52] This advice applies to any faith-based project. Business people often consider that non-profit organizations are too preoccupied with formulating their mission, but it is an essential task, 'because that is how a nonprofit builds a sense of community and shared values'.[53] Mission, not markets, is the primary magnet inspiring passion, loyalty and hard work from staff and volunteers.[54] It is the mission and its values that must drive all decision-making. Consequently, it will be necessary to establish systematic evaluation processes to guarantee that the business pole of the healthcare mythology (see Chapter 2) does not become the dominant factor in decisions.

---

51   See Arbuckle 2000, pp.141–149, and (1999) 'Mission and business: Resolving the tension.' *Health Progress 80*, 5, 22–24.

52   See Carol Taylor (2001) 'Roman Catholic health care identity and mission.' *Christian Bioethics 7*, 1, 29–30, 44–45.

53   McFarlan 1999, 77.

54   See Jeffrey L. Bradach, Thomas J. Tierney and Nan Stone (2008) 'Delivering on the promise of nonprofits.' *Harvard Business Review 86*, 12, 90–91.

Guideline 2: Institutions must have a 'preferential option for the poor'

The phrase, a 'preferential option for the poor', was developed by Catholic liberation theologians in the 1970s.[55] The theology behind this guideline has its roots in the scriptural understanding of the causes of poverty and its degrading impact on people's lives. It also assumes that the chief and conscious agents of liberation are people who are caught in the poverty trap. Others must cooperate, but in ways that foster this movement of the people in their own growth. The scriptural tradition, based on the Good Samaritan story, advocates that people have a right to healthcare services; they are not merely to be offered to people on the margins of society from the financial surplus of an institution, but from its capital, if necessary.[56] The guideline does not exclude working with people who are not poor, but it does mean that, in decision-making, the trustees and boards of Catholic healthcare facilities must give especial emphasis to the needs of people who are poor.

Guideline 3: Develop inductive formation programmes for board members, executives and staff

There are three interconnected essential qualities of any institutional cultural identity: first, a founding or genesis story, that is, its founding myth. This fundamental myth inspires and empathetically tells people who they are, what is good and bad (see Chapter 1). Next are the visible markers of this myth, especially behaviours; and, finally, effective formal and informal processes are necessary to educate people about the founding story and the visible markers of a distinctive identity. If a culture does not have these adequate educational processes in place then its unique identity can never be maintained.

Every organization, including Catholic healthcare institutions, has the right to require its staff members to behave according to the tenets of its founding story, mission and values. This does not mean that they need to become Catholics, but there are certain non-

---

55   See Gustavo Gutierrez (1993) *A Theology of Liberation*. Maryknoll, NY: Orbis.
56   See Gerald A. Arbuckle (2007) *'A Preferential Option for the Poor': Application to Catholic Health and Aged Care Ministries in Australia*. Canberra: Catholic Health Australia, pp.52–57.

negotiables, such as the values of the Good Samaritan parable, that people must adhere to. Their behaviour based on these values will be the visible markers of the organization's identity. Hence, appropriate, experientially based formation programmes for all staff members are essential.

A distinction needs to be made between leadership development and leadership formation programmes. The former focus on developing business skills, but the latter emphasize training people in the vision, mission and values of faith-based institutions.[57] Formation programmes are to be based on the principles of adult learning. Ultimately, identity in non-profit healthcare today will be embedded only by dialogue and persuasion, not by dictates from above. Some of the biggest disasters in American industry, as educationalist Martha Nussbaum reminded us, have been due 'to a culture of yes-people, where authority and peer group pressure ruled the roost and critical ideas were never articulated'.[58] Faith-based healthcare must be prepared to invest in skilled educationalists. This may be a costly exercise, but without their professional expertise, the founding story of healthcare will not be creatively assimilated. They have the ability to build on people's experiences by using the Socratic question and answer method in order to stimulate participants' imagination and their ability to apply the mission creatively to changing circumstances.[59] Board members, senior executives and middle managers will need more extensive programmes than other staff members. It is increasingly common for board members and senior executives to participate in retreats at the sacred sites of the original founding order. Further, trustees, board members and senior executives are to be encouraged to participate in meaningful 'poverty exposure programmes' to discover experientially how people feel when they are socially and economically marginalized. This could mean, for example, acting as volunteer helpers for periods of time in services like soup kitchens or refugee centres. One extensive Catholic healthcare system in Australia has developed faith-based,

---

57   See John O. Mudd (2009) 'When knowledge and skill aren't enough: Leadership formation takes leaders to new levels.' *Health Progress 90*, 5, 26–32.

58   Martha C. Nussbaum (2011) *Not for Profit: Why Democracy Needs the Humanities.* Princeton, NJ: Princeton University Press, p.53.

59   Ibid., pp.47–77.

reflection-praxis groups within their facilities. They meet regularly to reflect on particular aspects of their vision and mission statements in the light of their experience as staff members. Practical action is planned as the result of their reflections. For example, the national board of this healthcare system gathers for an hour prior to their monthly meeting to undertake such reflection. Members claim that this reflective period positively influences the way they interact with one another in the formal board meeting that follows.

Guideline 4: Appoint appropriate people to key positions

The virtue of justice, along with excellence, as evident in the Good Samaritan parable, requires that staff members in Catholic healthcare facilities meet standards set out in their job description. Patients and the facilities themselves have the right to expect this. It is a misinterpretation of compassion for a facility to tolerate undue, repeated failures by staff members. The manner in which staff members are reminded of their obligations, however, will always be done in ways that respect their dignity as people.

This understanding of justice is important when it comes to employment of personnel in faith-based healthcare facilities. Nothing is more decisive to the achievement of patient and staff satisfaction than the personal beliefs of the trustees, board, senior executive and middle management. They must be passionate about the mission. There is nothing 'wrong' with experience and professional knowledge, but 'as not-for-profits have learned, there's a lot more right with passion'.[60] It is as simple as that. Historian George Marsden, reflecting on the history of some of America's universities and colleges that were formerly faith-based, concluded that once a faith-based 'institution adopts the policy that it will hire [people not committed the mission], it is simply a matter of time until its faculty will have an ideological profile essentially like that of the faculty at every other mainstream university'. He argued that the first loyalties of faculty staffs will be to the national cultures of their professions rather than to any local or ecclesiastical traditions. It is impossible to change this movement and this means that 'the church

---

60   Nancy Lublin (2010) *Zilch: The Power of Zero in Business*. London: Penguin, p.138.

tradition becomes vestigial'.[61] The comment is equally relevant to faith-based healthcare services.

In healthcare facilities the critically important people are sponsors, trustees, directors of boards, CEOs and key executives. However, the success of a healthcare facility in these turbulent times depends more on the creative ability, competence, and drive of the CEO than on any other individual.[62] The CEO, as delegated by the board, must ensure that the mission permeates all decision-making and action, and so must believe in the philosophy of Catholic healthcare. Barry Eisenberg commented on the importance of this point in healthcare organizations: 'Nothing is more critical to the achievement of customer service...than the personal beliefs of the senior executive and board. It's really that simple.'[63] These important personnel will need to be motivated, not only by Catholic healthcare values in their personal and professional lives, but they need to have ready access to the fundamental theological information that is the source of these values.

Guideline 5: Avoid the uncritical acceptance of management language

In recent times the language of non-profit healthcare administrations has changed significantly in favour of business management; for example, heads of hospitals are called 'chief executive officers'. Unless healthcare people are careful, they can be seduced into adopting the competitive and patriarchal assumptions of some management jargon. What Basil Mott, Dean of Health Studies, University of New Hampshire, wrote in 1986 still remains relevant today: 'I speak of such...tough talk as strategy, tactics, market penetration, and product realignment-jargon that depicts a world of winners and losers, a macho world that is like war.' This is scarcely 'a language that evokes the values of serving and caring for human beings'.[64] The values of

61   George Marsden, cited by Peter Steinfels (1995) 'Catholic identity: Emerging consensus.' *Origins 25*, 11, 175.

62   See John R. Katzenbach and Douglas K. Smith (1994) *The Wisdom of Teams*. New York: Harper-Business, p.45.

63   Barry Eisenberg (1997) 'Customer service in healthcare: A new era.' *Hospital and Health Service Administration 42*, 1, 25. See also Arbuckle 2000, pp.228–230.

64   Basil J. Mott (1986) 'Whither the soul of health care?' In Richard M.F. Southby and Warren Greenberg (eds) *The For-Profit Hospital*. Columbus, OH: Battelle Press, p.144.

faith-based healthcare, as they emerge in the Good Samaritan story, are diametrically opposed to this kind of patriarchal and competitive management language. We surely need well-researched strategies and targets, but they must always be prepared and implemented in the context of the mission of holistic healing.

Guideline 6: Avoid tribalism

One certain sign that economic rationalism has invaded faith-based healthcare would be the emergence of tribalism between systems. Divisive tribalism strikes at the very heart of solidarity, which is an integral quality inherent in the Good Samaritan parable. When individual systems interiorize this quality of national solidarity, they will willingly collaborate across the boundaries of their systems for the general good of faith-based services. However, since Catholic healthcare systems have commonly acted very independently of each other, collaboration is not easy.

Guideline 7: Avoid an overemphasis on historical founding figures

Most Catholic healthcare or aged care facilities owe their origins to some founding person of a religious order that owns, or formerly owned, the facility. While the story of their founding of the order is important, it is no longer sufficient to sustain the facilities into the future, especially when mergers across once competitive boundaries inevitably becomes essential for survival and growth. Hence, the urgency to return to the story that forms the genesis of all individual facilities, that is, the Good Samaritan story. Moreover, even these individual foundation stories become very thin indeed unless they are constantly re-energized by reference to the ultimate founding story itself.

Guideline 8: Avoid 'addiction' to the mission

The language of mission can be used as an escape from reality. It becomes the 'good', and business becomes an 'evil of the profane world'. The mission is referred to and praised for its inspiring beauty, something 'holy', not to be polluted through contact with the profane world of 'the business'. This false theology is as destructive as an overemphasis on business management. Anne Schaef and Diane Fassel have shown that the exaltation of the mission and the downplaying of business realities can be a form of addiction for a group. Administrators and employees can 'become hooked on the promise of the mission and choose not to look at how the system is operating'. The failings of the healthcare facility are dismissed 'because [the latter] has a lofty mission'.[65] The noble language of organization's mission statement is used to hide the injustices and bad business practices in the facilities.

Guideline 9: Faith-based initiatives, whereby governments and faith-based institutions formally collaborate in healthcare projects, can significantly benefit the community, provided safeguards are in place to protect the identity of the latter

Before signing contracts with a government, faith-based organizations must be certain that the new partner understands their mission and values, accepts them as equals and acknowledges that the primary focus of the joint projects is the welfare of people, not the short-term political advantage of a government. The contract will include structures that ensure mutual accountability.

Summary

○ Faith-based organizations are significantly religious in nature and generally non-profit, as compared to commercial, government or private secular institutions. Over the centuries these organizations have had a profoundly positive impact on the development of healthcare services, particularly emphasizing the needs of people who are poor.

○ These institutions are now threatened by dramatically rising financial costs and changing social values. They must find ways to maintain their mission of holistic healing as the driving

---

65   Anne W. Schaef and Diane Fassel (1990) *The Addictive Organization*. San Francisco, CA: Harper & Row, p.123.

force in all decision-making. Partnering with governments in healthcare services can have beneficial results for all involved, but there are serious risks unless contractual safeguards are in place.

○ There are three interconnected essential qualities of any institutional cultural identity: first, a founding or genesis story, that is, its founding myth; second, the visible markers of identity, especially behaviours; and finally, the formal and informal educational processes of the founding story and the visible identity makers of distinctiveness must remain firmly in place. Ongoing educational formation of their staff is an essential requirement for maintaining the faith-based identity of these institutions. The emphasis is on imbuing staff at every institutional level with a clear, passionate 'sense of purpose and a belief that their individual actions will help realize the overall goal'.[66] The behaviour of an individual or a group is actually the defining mark of who they are.

Strategic implications

Policies

○ Since 'the mission' and not 'the business ethic' must be the guiding force in the formulation of all policies and decision-making for faith-based healthcare organizations, their trustees and members of the governing boards must ensure that the founding story and its values are known and firmly embedded in their cultures. This cannot be achieved unless they themselves are informed of, and transformed by, the mission and values that are integral to their founding story.

Implementation

○ Only people who are prepared to be attitudinally and operationally deeply imbued by the mission and values of the organization should be appointed to key positions, including senior and middle management staff.

---

66   Lublin 2010, p.14.

○ Since the CEO has been delegated authority from the trustees and board to make sure the mission and values are inculcated within the organizational culture, it is particularly important that the CEO has the right qualities to lead a faith-based healthcare facility.

○ Normally the CEO in a faith-based institutions operationally delegates a particular official, often termed the *mission leader*, with the task of ensuring that staff members know, accept and are transformed by its mission and values. Since mission leaders primarily have personal authority, not position or executive authority, they need to be able to understand the pressures and tensions of the business side of healthcare facilities, as well as having gifts of communication and creativity, in order to be credible and effective in this role.[67] They need to be publicly supported by the board and administration, and provided with adequate resources to fulfil their central role in the institution.

---

67 In a survey conducted in 2006 in the USA, respondents ranked the following skills the most important: ability to work well in a team; good oral communication skills; group facilitation skills; knowledge of business practice; labor relation skills; and written communication gifts. See Patricia A. Talone (2006) 'CHA mission leaders survey.' *Health Progress 87*, 2, 20.

Discussion Questions

Chapter 1: Power and Complexity of Culture: Healthcare Insights

1. What insights do you find in this chapter that are particularly helpful in understanding the culture of your workplace?

2. What do you perceive to be the symbols of power in your workplace culture/subculture? Do you feel they are being used in the best interests of staff and patients?

3. What are the myths or stories that bind your workplace culture together? Who are the cultural heroes and the effective storytellers in your culture/subculture?

4. What periods of chaos have you had in your life? What did you feel? What did you learn from them? Have there been, or are there at present, organizational cultural chaos experiences at your workplace? How do you perceive how you yourself and the management are coping with them?

5. In your healthcare facility what is being done that positively respects the cultural diversity of patients?

Chapter 2: Healthcare Models in Conflict: What about the Patient?

1. In your healthcare facility what healthcare model do you think predominantly controls policies and their implementation? What are reasons for your answer? How do others in your workplace answer these questions?

2. As the Good Samaritan story is historically the residual founding myth of healthcare in the Western world, what values in the story are operative in your workplace? What

values are not, but should be, operative, and what do you think you could do personally to embed these values in your workplace culture?

3. There will always be a tension in healthcare facilities between the foundational mission and values of healthcare and the need to remain financially viable. What are the mechanisms in place to guarantee that the mission/values are driving all decision-making? What structures are needed to maintain the mission/values as the senior partner in the tension?

Chapter 3: Tribalism between Clinicians and Managers: Risk to Patients

1. Stereotypes are preformed images or pictures that we have of things or people; they are shorthand, but faulty, methods of handling, grasping and controlling a complex cultural world. As they encourage us to prejudge people of other cultures, what stereotypes does your subculture have of other subcultures in your workplace? The stereotypes that managers carry of clinicians? Clinicians of managers?

2. What practical steps could you individually, and the group you work with, take to get to know personally people of other subcultures in your healthcare institution? What values in the foundational story of healthcare should motivate you and your group in this task?

Chapter 4: Bullying in Healthcare Institutions: An Anthropological Perspective

1. Does your organization have a code of ethics that forbids bullying? If not, what can you do to pressure management to introduce such a code? If your organization does have a code, are there examples where it is not being upheld?

2. Give an example of a whistleblower who uncovered bullying incidents in your institution? How was that person treated by

their colleagues and by management? How could you have helped to support the person?

3. Identify an experience where you were bullied. What did you feel? What did you learn from the experience? What advice would you offer a victim as result of your experience?

4. Individually or in groups, identify examples where your organizational culture is encouraging or tolerating bullying behaviour towards individuals or groups of people? What would you do to alert management to this abusive behaviour?

Chapter 5: Leading Cultural Change in Healthcare

1. In your experience can you identify a paramodern leader? What are the qualities that particularly characterized their behaviour?

2. If you are a manager, what should you do to encourage paramodern leaders at all levels of your healthcare organization? Do you celebrate their achievements within your organizational culture? If not, how could you do this?

3. What are the gaps (if any) between the mission and the reality of your healthcare? What do you feel about these gaps? How would you and your colleagues go about bridging these gaps?

Chapter 6: Leading Mergers in Healthcare: Cultural Processes

1. Have you personally experienced an example of an organizational merger? What did you feel and learn about this experience? How did management lead the process? In retrospect, what would you have done if you had the task of leading the process?

2. In your experience of restructuring, how have managers respected the foundational values of your healthcare institution in relating to staff members?

3. Imagine that you are in the midst of a merger with another healthcare subculture. What could you do personally or as a manager to ritualize the stages of the process?

Chapter 7: Faith-Based Healthcare: A Case Study

1. Since the unique identity of a faith-based healthcare is the actual day-to-day living out of the mission and values of its founding story at all levels of the organizational culture, what educational, transformative processes are in place to ensure the story is known and constantly evaluated for its effectiveness?

2. As a trustee or board member identify a particular decision that has been made. At what stage and to what extent, if at all, were the options evaluated in light of the mission and values?

3. Imagine as a trustee or board member you are concerned that the senior executive is not acting according to the organization's mission and values. What are your obligations? How would you discover what is happening and rectify, if necessary, the situation?

4. Since the founding story is kept alive by example of individuals and groups, what can you do to record and publish the stories of their example?

5. By identifying and responding to community needs, faith-based healthcare institutions are living out their foundational mission and values by demonstrating their concern for human dignity and the poor and vulnerable in society. Is this actually happening in your institution? If not, what can you do to ensure that 'the mission' is driving 'the business' in decision-making?

Further Reading

Chapter 1: Power and Complexity of Culture: Healthcare Insights

Armstrong, D. (2002) *A New History of Identity: A Sociology of Medical Knowledge*. Basingstoke: Palgrave Macmillan.

Barnard, A. (2000) *History and Theory in Anthropology*. Cambridge: Cambridge University Press.

Mannion, R., Davies, H. and Marshall, M. (2004) *Cultures for Performance*. Buckingham: Open University Press.

Pool, R. and Geissler, W. (2005) *Medical Anthropology*. Maidenhead: Open University Press.

Chapter 2: Healthcare Models in Conflict: What about the Patient?

Dickinson, H. and Mannion, R. (eds) (2011) *The Reform of Health Care: Shaping, Adapting and Resisting Policy Developments*. Basingstoke: Palgrave Macmillan.

Klein, R. (2006) *The New Politics of the NHS*, 5th edn. Abingdon: Radcliffe Publishing.

Palmer, G.R. and Ho, M.T. (2008) *Health Economics: A Critical Global Analysis*. Basingstoke: Palgrave Macmillan.

Pattison, S., Hannigan, B., Pill, R. and Thomas, H. (2010) *Emerging Values in Health Care*. London: Jessica Kingsley Publishers.

Chapter 3: Tribalism between Clinicians and Managers: Risk to Patients

Degeling, P., Sorrenson, R., Aisbett, C., Zhang, K. and Coyle, B. (2000) *The Organisation of Hospital Care and its Effects*. Sydney: Centre for Hospital Management and Information Systems Research.

Gopee, N. and Galloway, J. (2009) *Leadership and Management in Healthcare*. London: Sage Publications.

Kets de Vries, M.F. and Miller, D. (1985) *The Neurotic Organization*. San Francisco, CA: Jossey-Bass.

Parkin, P. (2009) *Managing Change in Healthcare: Using Action Research*. London: Sage Publications.

Chapter 4: Bullying in Healthcare Institutions: An Anthropological Perspective

Namie, G. and Namie, R. (2000) *The Bully at Work*. Naperville, IL: Sourcebooks.

Rigby, K. (2002) *New Perspectives on Bullying*. London: Jessica Kingsley Publishers.

Riley, D., Duncan, D.J. and Edwards, J. (2012) *Bullying of Staff in Schools*. Camberwell: Australian Council for Educational Research.

Salin, D. (2003) *Workplace Bullying among Business Professionals: Prevalence, Organisational Antecedents and Gender Differences*. Helsinki: Yliopistopaino, Helsingfors.

Chapter 5: Leading Cultural Change in Healthcare

Byock, I. (2012) *The Best Care Possible: A Physician's Quest to Transform Care Through the End of Life*. New York: Avery.

Engel, J.D., Zarconi, J., Pethtel, L.L. and Missimi, S.A. (2008) *Narrative in Health Care*. Abingdon: Radcliffe Publishing.

Loughlin, M. (2002) *Ethics, Management and Mythology*. Abingdon: Radical Medical Press.

Storey, J., Bullivant, J. and Corbett-Nolan, A. (2011) *Governing the New NHS: Issues and Tensions in Health Service Management*. Abingdon: Routledge.

Wenneberg, J.E. (2010) *Tracking Medicine: A Researcher's Quest to Understand Health Care*. New York: Oxford University Press.

Chapter 6: Leading Mergers in Healthcare: Cultural Processes

Habeck, M.M., Kroger, F. and Tram, M.R. (2000) *After the Merger*. London: Prentice Hall.

Hartley, J. and Benington, J. (2010) *Leadership for Healthcare*. Bristol: Policy Press.

Turner, V. (1974) *Dramas, Fields, and Metaphors: Symbolic Action in Human Society*. Ithaca, NY: Cornell University Press.

Wall, J. and Wall, S.R. (2000) *The Morning After: Making Corporate Mergers Work after the Deal is Sealed*. Cambridge, MA: Perseus Publishing.

Chapter 7: Faith-Based Healthcare: A Case Study

Arbuckle, G.A. (2000) *Healthcare Ministry: Refounding the Mission in Tumultuous Times*. Collegeville, MN: Liturgical Press.

Mele D. (2009) *Business Ethics in Action: Seeking Human Excellence in Organizations*. Basingstoke: Palgrave Macmillan.

Nelson, L.J. (2009) *Diagnosis: The Urgent Threats Confronting Catholic Health Care*. Huntington, IN: Our Sunday Visitor.

Wall, B.M. (2011) *American Catholic Hospitals: A Century of Changing Markets and Mission*. New Brunswick, NJ: Rutgers University Press.

REFERENCES

Academy of Royal Medical Colleges and NHS Institute (2007) *Enhancing Engagement in Medical Leadership.* Available at www.institute.nhs.uk.

Ackerman, P. and Duvall, J. (2000) *A Force More Powerful: A Century of Nonviolent Conflict.* New York: Palgrave Macmillan.

Adams, A. (1992) *Bullying at Work.* London: Virago Press.

Adams, D. (1960) 'The monkey and the fish: Cultural pitfalls of an educational adviser.' *International Development Review 2,* 2.

Alford, C.F. (1995) 'The group as a whole or acting out the missing leader.' *International Journal of Group Psychotherapy 45,* 1.

Allport, G. (1958) *The Nature of Prejudice.* New York: Doubleday.

Allsop, J. (1995) *Health Policy and the NHS: Towards 2000.* London: Longman.

'American health care.' (1998) *The Economist* (7 March), 21–24.

Anderson, C., Bishop, M., Cairncross, F., Carson, I. *et al.* (2000) *Making Mergers Work.* London: The Economist.

Anderson, W.T. (1995) *The Truth about Truth: De-confusing and Re-constructing the Postmodern World.* New York: Putnam.

Annandale, E. (1998) *The Sociology of Health and Medicine: A Critical Introduction.* Oxford: Polity Press.

Arbuckle, G.A. (1991) *Grieving for Change.* London: Geoffrey Chapman.

Arbuckle, G.A. (1993) *Refounding the Church; Dissent for Leadership.* Maryknoll, NY: Orbis.

Arbuckle, G.A. (1999) 'Mission and business: Resolving the tension.' *Health Progress 80,* 5, 22–24.

Arbuckle, G.A. (2000) *Healthcare Ministry: Refounding the Mission in Tumultuous Times.* Collegeville, MN: Liturgical Press.

Arbuckle, G.A. (2003) *Dealing with Bullies.* London: St Pauls Publishing.

Arbuckle, G.A. (2004) *Violence, Society, and the Church: A Cultural Approach.* Collegeville, MN: Liturgical Press.

Arbuckle, G.A. (2007) '*A Preferential Option for the Poor': Application to Catholic Health and Aged Care Ministries in Australia.* Canberra: Catholic Health Australia.

Arbuckle, G.A. (2010) *Culture, Inculturation, and Theologians: A Postmodern Critique.* Collegeville, MN: Liturgical Press.

Armstrong, P. and Armstrong, H. (1998) *Universal Healthcare.* New York: New Press.

Auerbach, A., Landefeld, C.S. and Shojania, K.G. (2007) 'The tension between needing to improve care and knowing how to do it.' *New England Journal of Medicine 357,* 6.

Bader, B.S. (1977) 'Look before you leap: Boards need to ask "why?" before merging or affiliating.' *Trustee 50,* 3.

'Balancing broomsticks.' (1994) *The Economist* (25 June), 85.

Bargh, J.A. and Alvarez, J. (2001) 'The Road to Hell: Good Intentions in the Face of Unconscious Tendencies to Misuse Power.' In A.Y. Lee-Chai and J.A. Bargh (eds) *The Use and Abuse of Power.* New York: New York University Press.

Barnard, A. (2000) *History and Theory in Anthropology.* Cambridge: Cambridge University Press.

Barthes, R. (1982) 'Introduction to the Structural Analysis of Narratives.' In Susan Sontag (ed.) *A Barthes Reader.* London: Cape.

Bate, P. (1994) *Strategies for Cultural Change.* Oxford: Butterworth-Heinemann.

Batson, C.D. (1975) 'Attribution as a mediator of bias in helping.' *Journal of Personality and Social Psychology 32,* 3.

Beal, J.P. (1994) 'Catholic hospitals: How Catholic will they be?' *Concilium 5,* 89.

Bennis, W. (1989) *On Becoming a Leader.* Reading, MA: Addison-Wesley.

Berger, P. (1969) *The Sacred Canopy: Elements of a Sociological Theory of Religion.* New York: Doubleday.

Berger, P. (1974) *Pyramids of Sacrifice: Political Ethics and Social Change.* Harmondsworth: Penguin.

Berwick, D.M. (2009) 'What "patient-centered" should mean: Confessions of an extremist.' *Health Affairs 28,* 4.

Bion, W. (1967) *Second Thoughts.* London: Heinemann.

Black-Michard, J. (1975) *Feuding Societies*. Oxford: Basil Blackwell.
Blane, D. (1997) 'Health Professions.' In Graham Scambler (ed.) *Sociology as Applied to Medicine*, 4th edn. London: W.B. Saunders.
Block, P. (1993) *Stewardship: Choosing Service over Self-Interest*. San Francisco, CA: Berrett-Koehler.
Bocock, R. (1974) *Ritual in Industrial Society: A Sociological Analysis of Ritualism in Modern England*. London: George Allen and Unwin.
Boston, J. and Dalziel, P. (1992) *The Decent Society?* Oxford: Oxford University Press.
Bowlby, J. (1980) *Loss: Sadness and Depression*. New York: Basic Books.
Bradach, J.L., Tierney, T.J. and Stone, N. (2008) 'Delivering on the promise of nonprofits.' *Harvard Business Review 86*, 12, 90–91.
Bridges, W. (1995) *Jobshift*. London: Nicholas Brealey Publishing.
British Medical Association (BMA) (1997) *BMA Annual Report of Council 1996–97*. London: BMA.
British Medical Association (BMA) (2009) 'Whistleblowing: Advice for BMA Members Working in Secondary Care about Raising Concerns in the Workplace.' Accessed on 3/3/10 at www.bma.org. uk/Whistleblowing.ashx.
Bristol Royal Infirmary Inquiry (2001) *Learning from Bristol: The Report of the Public Inquiry into Children's Heart Surgery at the Bristol Royal Infirmary 1984–1995*. Accessed on 12/6/12 at www.bristol-inquiry. org.uk.
Brooker, P. (1999) *A Concise Glossary of Cultural Theory*. London: Arnold.
Brooks, D. (2011) *The Social Animal: The Hidden Sources of Love, Character, and Achievement*. New York: Random House.
Brophy, M. (2011) 'Study: ERs shrink as demand rises.' *USA Today* (17 May), 8.
Broyles, W. (1986) 'A ritual for saying goodbye.' *US News and World Report* (10 November).
Buber, M. (2002) *Between Man and Man*. New York: Routledge.
Buchanan, M. (1998) 'Fascinating rhythm.' *New Scientist 157*, 215, 20–25.
Buck, P. (1958) *The Coming of the Maori*. Wellington, NZ: Whitcombe and Tombs.
Bureau of Health Information (2010) *Insights into Care: Patients' Perspectives on NSW Public Hospitals*. Sydney: NSW Government.
Burns, J.M. (1978) *Leadership*. New York: Harper Torch.
Burtchaell, J.T. (1998) *The Dying of the Light: The Disengagement of Colleges and Universities from their Christian Churches*. Grand Rapids, MN: William B. Eerdmans.
Butler, J. (1999) *The Ethics of Health Care Rationing: Principles and Practices*. London: Cassell.
Byrne, B. (2000) *The Hospitality of God: A Reading of Luke's Gospel*. Sydney: St Pauls Publications.
Cahill, P. (1994) 'Collaboration among Catholic health providers.' *Origins 24*, 12.
Callahan, D. (1998) *False Hopes: Why America's Quest for Perfect Health is a Recipe for Failure*. New York: Simon & Schuster.
Callahan, D. (2009) *Taming the Beloved Beast: How Medical Technology Costs are Destroying Our Health Care System*. Princeton, NJ: Princeton University Press.
Campbell, J. (1949) *The Hero with a Thousand Faces*. Princeton, NJ: Princeton University Press.
Campbell, J. (1970) *The Masks of God*, 4 vols. New York: Viking Press.
Campbell, S.M. (1995) *From Chaos to Confidence*. New York: Simon & Schuster.
Cartwright, S. and Cooper, C.L. (1993) 'The psychological impact of merger and acquisition on the individual.' *Human Relations 46*, 3, 327–329.
Casement, P.J. (1991) *Learning from the Patient*. New York: Guilford Press.
Castells, M. (1996) *The Power of Identity: Volume 2: The Information Age: Economy, Society and Culture*. Oxford: Blackwell.
'Catholic health care poised between mission and money.' (1998) *National Catholic Reporter* Editorial (23 January), 36.
Chan, J.B.L. (1997) *Changing Police Culture: Policing in a Multicultural Society*. Cambridge: Cambridge University Press.
Cheyne, C., O'Brien, M. and Belgrave, M. (2008) *Social Policy in Aotearoa New Zealand*, 4th edn. Melbourne: Oxford University Press.
Child, A.B. and Child, I.L. (1993) *Religion and Magic in the Life of Traditional Peoples*. Englewood Cliffs, NJ: Prentice Hall.
Clifton, G. (2009) 'Healing health care.' *America* (8–15 June).
Cogley, J. (1974) *Catholic America*. New York: Image.
Cohen, B. (1997) *The Edge of Chaos: Financial Booms, Bubbles, Crashes and Chaos*. Chichester: Wiley.
Cole, D. (2011) 'Health care reform unconstitutional?' *The New York Review* (24 February), 9–11.
Coleman, J.A. (1982) *An American Strategic Theology*. New York: Paulist.

Collini, S. (2012) *What Are Universities for?* London: Penguin.

Commission on Urban Life and Faith (2006) *Faithful Cities: A Call for Celebration, Vision and Justice.* Peterborough: Methodist Publishing House.

Conner, D.R. (1993) *Managing at the Speed of Change.* New York: Villard Books.

Cooper, Z., Gibbons, S., Jones, S. and McGuire, A. (2011) 'Does hospital competition save lives? Evidence from the English NHS Patient Choice Reforms.' *Economic Journal 121*, 554 (August), 228–260.

Coulter, A. (2005) 'The NHS revolution: Health care in the market place – what do patients and the public want from primary care?' *British Medical Journal 331* (19 November), 1199–1201.

Coutu, D.L. (2002) 'The anxiety of learning.' *Harvard Business Review 80*, 3.

Covey, S. (1990) *The Seven Habits of Highly Effective People: Powerful Lessons in Personal Change.* New York: Simon & Schuster.

Cox, D. (1992) 'Crisis and Opportunity in Health Service Management.' In R. Loveridge and K. Starkey (eds) *Continuity and Crisis in the NHS.* Buckingham: Open University Press.

Crinson, I. (2009) *Health Policy: A Critical Perspective.* London: Sage Publications.

Crosson, F.J. (2003) 'Kaiser Permanente: A propensity for partnership.' *British Medical Journal 326* (22 March).

Curran, C.E. (1997) 'The Catholic identity of Catholic institutions.' *Theological Studies 58*, 1, 90–108.

Dagan, H. (1999) 'In defense of the Good Samaritan.' *Michigan Law Review 97*, 5.

Dante Alighieri (1909) *The Divine Comedy,* trans. H.W. Longfellow. New York: Doubleday.

Dash, P. and Meredith, D. (2010) 'When and how provider competition can improve health care delivery.' *McKinsey Quarterly.* Accessed at www.mckinseyquarterly.com.

Davies, D.J. (2011) *Emotion, Identity, and Religion: Hope, Reciprocity, and Otherness.* Oxford: Oxford University Press.

Davies, H.T.O. and Harrison, S. (2003) 'Trends in doctor–manager relationships.' *British Medical Journal 326* (22 March).

Davies, H.T.O., Hodges, C.-L. and Rundall, T.G. (2003) 'Views of doctors and managers on doctor–manager relationship in the NHS.' *British Medical Journal 326* (22 March), 626–628.

Davis, F., Paulhus, E. and Bradstock, A. (2008) *Moral, but No Compass: Government, Church and the Future of the Welfare State.* Chelmsford: Mathew James.

Deacon, A. (2008) 'Employment.' In P. Alcock, M. May and K. Rowlingson (eds) *The Student's Companion to Social Policy.* Oxford: Blackwell.

Deal, T.E. and Kennedy, A.A. (1982) *Corporate Cultures: The Rites and Rituals of Corporate Life.* Reading, MA: Addison-Wesley.

Dees, J.G. (1999) 'Enterprising Nonprofits.' In *Harvard Business Review on Nonprofits.* Boston, MA: Harvard Business School Publishing.

Degeling, P. and Carr, A. (2004) 'Leadership for the systemization of health care: The unaddressed issue in health care reform.' *Journal of Health Organization and Management 18*, 6, 399–414.

Degeling, P., Maxwell, S., Kennedy, J. and Coyle, B. (2003) 'Medicine, management, and modernization: A "danse macabre"?' *British Medical Journal 326* (22 March), 649–652.

Dekker, S. (2007) *Just Culture: Balancing Safety and Accountability.* Farnham: Ashgate.

Deloitte Center for Health Solutions (2010) *Issue Brief: Social Networks in Health Care: Communication, Collaboration and Insights 1,* 4. Accessed 15/8/11 at www.deloitte.com/NS_CHS_2010SocialNetworks_070710.pdf.

Denning, S. (2001) *The Springboard: How Storytelling Ignites Action in Knowledge-Era Organizations.* Boston, MA: Butterworth-Heinemann.

Department of Health (DoH) (1998) *A First Class Service: Quality in the New NHS.* London: DoH.

Department of Health (DoH) (2000a) *An Organisation with a Memory.* London: DoH.

Department of Health (DoH) (2000b) *The NHS Plan: A Plan for Investment, A Plan for Reform.* London: Stationery Office.

Department of Health (2003) *Tackling Health Inequalities: A Programme for Action.* London: DoH.

Department of Health (DoH) (2004) *The NHS Improvement Plan: Putting People at the Heart of Public Services.* London: Stationery Office.

Department of Health (DoH) (2005) *Creating a Patient-Led NHS: Developing the NHS Improvement Plan.* London: DoH.

Department of Health (2010) *Equity and Excellence: Liberating the NHS.* London: DoH.

Department of Health and Social Security (DoH) (1988) *Community Care: Agenda for Action* (Griffiths Report). London: HMSO.

Department of Social Security (1950) *The Growth and Development of Social Security in New Zealand.* Wellington, NZ: Government Printer.

Descartes, R. (1996) *Discourse on the Method and Meditations on First Philosophy*, ed. D. Weissman, trans. E. Haldane and G.R. Ross. New Haven, CT: Yale University Press.

Dolan, S., Garcia, S. and Richley, B. (2006) *Managing by Values*. Basingstoke: Palgrave Macmillan.

Douglas, M. (1966) *Purity and Danger: An Analysis of the Concepts of Pollution and Taboo*. London: Routledge & Kegan Paul.

Douglas, M. (1970) *Natural Symbols: Explorations in Cosmology*. New York: Pantheon Books.

Douglas, M. (1978) *Cultural Bias*. London: Royal Anthropological Institute.

Dow, D.A. (1995) *Safeguarding the Public Health: A History of the New Zealand Department of Health*. Wellington, NZ: Victoria University Press.

Drife, J. and Johnston, I. (1995) 'Handling the conflicting cultures in the NHS.' *British Medical Journal 310* (22 April), 1054–1056.

Drucker, P. (1982) *Managing in Turbulent Times*. London: Pan Books.

Drucker, P. (1986) *Innovation and Entrepreneurship: Practice and Principles*. New York: Harper & Row.

Drucker, P. (1990) *Managing the Nonprofit Organization: Practices and Principles*. New York: HarperCollins.

'Drugs and medical errors killing one of every five Australians.' (2009) *Best Health*. Accessed 14/6/12 at www.besthealth.com.au/drugs-and-medical-errors-killing-one-of-every-five-australians.

Duckett, S. (2001) 'Does it matter who owns health facilities?' *Journal of Health Services Research and Policy 6*, 1, 59–62.

Dunbar, J., Reddy, P. and May, S. (2011) *Deadly Healthcare*. Bowen Hills, Queensland: Australian Academic Press.

Duncan, W.J., Ginter, P.M. and Swayne, L.E. (1995) *Strategic Management of Health Care Organizations*, 2nd edn. Oxford: Blackwell.

Durkheim, E. (1965) *The Rules of Sociological Method*, trans. S. Solovay and J. Mueller. New York: Free Press.

Dworkin, D. (2012) 'Why the mandate is constitutional: The real argument.' *New York Review of Books 59*, 8.

Dwyer, R.J. (2008) 'Benchmarking as a process for demonstrating organizational trustworthiness?' *Management Decision 46*, 8, 1211–1212.

Editorial (18 January 2011) *The Times*.

'Editorial Hospital pass.' (2011) *The Times* (17 January), 2.

Edwards, N., Kornack, M.J. and Silversin, J. (2002) 'Unhappy doctors: What are the causes and what can be done?' *British Medical Journal 324* (6 April), 835–838.

Edwards, N., Marshall, M., McLellan, A. and Abbasi, K. (2003) 'Doctors and managers: A problem without a solution?' *British Medical Journal 326* (22 March).

Eisenberg, B. (1997) 'Customer service in healthcare: A new era.' *Hospital and Health Service Administration 42*, 1.

Engel, J.D., Zarconi, J., Pethtel, L.L. and Missimi, S.A. (2008) *Narrative Health Care: Healing Patients, Practitioners, Profession, and Community*. Abingdon: Radcliffe Publishing.

Ernst & Young and Miller, B. (eds) (1994) *Mergers and Acquisitions: Back-to-Basics Techniques for the '90s*, 2nd edn. New York: John Wiley.

Evans-Pritchard, E.E. (1937) *Witchcraft Oracles and Magic among the Azande*. Oxford: Clarendon Press.

Farnsley, A.E. (2007) 'Faith-Based Initiatives.' In J.A. Beckford and N.J. Demerath (eds) *The Sage Handbook of the Sociology of Religion*. London: Sage Publications.

Fawcett, T. (1970) *The Symbolic Language of Religion*. London: SCM Press.

Fernando, S. (1991) *Mental Health, Race and Culture*. London: Macmillan.

Ferngren, G.B. (2009) *Medicine and Health Care in Early Christianity*. Baltimore, MD: Johns Hopkins University Press.

Field, J. and Peck, E. (2003) 'Mergers and acquisitions in the private sector: What are the lessons for health and social services?' *Social Policy and Administration 37*, 7, 742–755.

Fitzsimmons, P. and White, A. (1997) 'Medicine and management: A conflict facing general practice.' *Journal of Management in Medicine 11*, 3, 124–131.

Flin, R. (2010) 'Rudeness at work: A threat to patient safety and quality of care.' *British Medical Journal 341* (31 July), 212–213.

Foster, D. (2010) *Research Brief: Differences in Health Quality Performance by Ownership*. Thomson Reuters, 9 August. Accessed 10/8/10 at www.100tophospitals.com/assets/100TopSystemOwnership.pdf.

Foster, G. (2010) *Study of the Response by Faith-Based Organizations to Orphans and Vulnerable Children – Preliminary Summary Report*, UNICEF. Accessed 18 June 2012 at www.jlica.org/pdf/unicefwrcpstudy.pdf.

Foster, G.M. (1972) 'The anatomy of envy: A study in symbolic behavior.' *Current Anthropology 13*, 2, 23–29.

Foucault, M. (1965) *Madness and Civilization: The History of Insanity in the Age of Reason*. New York: Random House.

Foucault, M. (1974) *The Order of Things: An Archaeology of the Human Sciences*. New York: Vintage Books.

Foucault, M. (1975) *The Birth of the Clinic: An Archaeology of Medical Perception*. New York: Vintage Books.

Foucault, M. (1979a) *Discipline and Punish: The Birth of the Prison*. Harmondsworth: Penguin.

Foucault, M. (1979b) *The History of Sexuality, Volume 1: An Introduction*. Harmondsworth: Penguin.

Francis, R. (2010) *Final Report of the Independent Inquiry by the Mid Staffordshire NHS Foundation Trust*. London: Stationery Office.

Freire, P. (1971) *Pedagogy of the Oppressed*. Harmondsworth: Penguin.

Freudenheim, M. (2000) 'Aetna to shed customers and jobs in effort to cut health care costs.' *The New York Times* (19 December), A1.

Friedman, E. (1996) 'Capitation, integration, and managed care.' *Journal of the American Medical Association 275*, 12.

Fromm, E. (1960)*The Fear of Freedom*. London: Routledge & Kegan Paul.

Fuchs, V. (1994) *The Future of Health Policy*. Cambridge, MA: Harvard University Press.

Fuhriman, A. and Burlingame, G.M. (1994) 'Measuring small group process: A methodological application of chaos theory.' *Small Group Research 25*, 4.

Fukuyama, F. (1995) *Trust: The Social Virtues and the Creation of Prosperity*. London: Hamish Hamilton.

Fuller Torrey, E. (1972) *Witchdoctors and Psychiatrists: The Common Roots of Psychology and Its Future*. New York: Harper & Row.

Furedi, F. (1998) *Culture of Fear: Risk-taking and the Morality of Low Expectation*. London: Cassell.

Galanti, G.-A. (1997) *Caring for Patients from Different Cultures: Case Studies from American Hospitals*, 2nd edn. Philadelphia, PA: University of Pennsylvania Press.

Garling, P. (2008a) *Final Report of the Special Commission of Inquiry Acute Care Services in NSW Public Hospitals, Vol. 1, Special Commission of Inquiry*. Sydney: NSW Government.

Garling, P. (2008b) *Final Report of the Special Commission of Inquiry: Acute Care Services in NSW Public Hospitals: Overview*. Sydney: NSW Government.

Gauld, R. (2009) *Revolving Doors: New Zealand's Health Reforms – The Continuing Saga*. Wellington, NZ: Health Services Research.

Geertz, C. (1973) *The Interpretation of Cultures*. New York: Basic Books.

Geertz, C. (1995) *After the Fact*. Cambridge, MA: Harvard University Press.

Gellner, E. (1992) *Postmodernism, Reason and Religion*. London: Routledge.

George, W.W. (2002) 'Imbalance of power.' *Harvard Business Review 80*, 7.

Germov, J. (1998) 'Challenges to Medical Dominance.' In J. Germov (ed.) *Second Opinion: An Introduction to Health Sociology*. Melbourne: Oxford University Press.

Giddens, A. (1990) *The Consequences of Modernity*. Cambridge: Polity Press.

Giddens, A. (1991) *Modernity and Self-Identity: Self and Society in the Late Modern Age*. Cambridge: Polity Press.

Giddens, A. (1992) *The Transformation of Intimacy: Sexuality, Love and Eroticism in Modern Societies*. Cambridge: Polity Press.

Glasser, J. (2011) 'Keep formation in-house.' *Health Progress 92*, 5.

Glazer, M.P. (1996) 'Ten Whistleblowers.' In M.D. Erman and R.J. Lundman (eds) *Corporate and Governmental Deviance*. New York: Oxford University Press.

Gleason, P. (1995) *Contending with Modernity: Catholic Higher Education in the Twentieth Century*. New York: Oxford University Press.

Glieck, J. (1987) *Chaos: Making a New Science*. New York: Penguin.

Gluckman, M. (1963) 'Gossip and scandal.' *Current Anthropology 4*, 4.

Goddard, M. and Ferguson, B. (1997) *Mergers in NHS: Made in Heaven or Marriages of Convenience*. London: Nuffield Trust.

Goldman, D. (2006) 'System failure versus personal accountability – the case for clean hands.' *New England Journal of Medicine 355*, 2, 121–123.

Goldsmith, A.J. (2000) 'An Impotent Conceit: Law, Culture and the Regulation of Police Violence.' In A. Coady, S. James, S. Miller and M. O'Keefe (eds) *Violence and Police Culture*. Melbourne: Melbourne University Press.

Goldsmith, S. (2010) *The Power of Social Innovation*. San Francisco, CA: Jossey-Bass.

Goodman, R.A. (1971) 'Some *Aitu* beliefs of modern Samoans.' *Journal of the Polynesian Society 80*, 4.

Gorer, G. (1965) *Death, Grief and Mourning*. London: Crescent Press.

Gornall, J. (2009) 'The price of silence.' *British Medical Journal 339* (31 October), 1000–1004.

Grace, G. (2002) *Catholic Schools: Mission, Markets and Morality*. London: RoutledgeFalmer.

Greener, I. (2009) *Healthcare in the UK: Understanding Continuity and Change*. Bristol: Policy Press.

Greenleaf, R.K. (1977) *Servant Leadership: A Journey into the Nature of Legitimate Power and Greatness*. New York: Paulist.

Greer, S.L. (2009) *The Politics of European Union Health Policies*. Maidenhead: Open University Press.

Grieg, A., Lewins, F. and White, K. (2003) *Inequality in Australia*. Cambridge: Cambridge University Press.

Groundwater-Smith, S. and Sachs, J. (2002) 'The activist professional and the reinstatement of trust.' *Cambridge Journal of Education 32*, 3, 67–84.

Gutierrez, G. (1973) *A Theology of Liberation*. Maryknoll, NY: Orbis.

Gvender, V. and Penn-Kekana, L. 'Gender biases and discrimination.' Geneva: World Health Organization. Accessed 25/8/11 at www.who.int/gender_biases_and_discrimination_wgkn_2007.pdf.

Hadikin, R. and O'Driscoll, M. (2000) *The Bullying Culture*. Oxford: Butterworth-Heinemann.

Hall, E.T. (1959) *The Silent Language*. New York: Doubleday Anchor.

Hall, E.T. (1986) *Beyond Culture*. New York: Doubleday/Anchor.

Ham, C. (2009) *Health Policy in Britain*. Basingstoke: Palgrave Macmillan.

Handler, J.F. and Hasenfeld, Y. (2007) *Blame Welfare, Ignore Poverty and Inequality*. Cambridge: Cambridge University Press.

Hands, D. (2010) 'Inspiration, Ideology, Evidence and the National Health.' Lecture to the Welsh Institute for Health and Social Care (9 March), p. 8. Accessed at www.sochealth.co.uk.

Handy, C. (1977) 'Unimagined Futures.' In M. Goldsmith, F. Hesselbein and R. Beckhard (eds) *The leader of the Future*. San Francisco, CA: Jossey-Bass.

Handy, C. (1985) *Understanding Voluntary Organizations*. London: Penguin.

Hann, C. (2000) *Social Anthropology*. Abingdon: Teach Yourself.

Harrison, S. and McDonald, R. (2008) *The Politics of Healthcare in Britain*. London: Sage Publications.

Hart, J.T. (2006) *The Political Economy of Health Care: A Clinical Perspective*. Bristol: Policy Press.

Hartford, T. (2011) *Adapt: Why Success Always Starts with Failure*. New York: Farrar, Strauss and Giroux.

Hartley, J. and Benington, J. (2010) *Leadership for Healthcare*. Bristol: Policy Press.

'Health care in America.' (2012) *The Economist* (4 February).

'Health insurance.' (1997) *The Economist* (13 December).

'Health reforms under attack.' (2011) *The Economist* (20 August), 32.

Heap, J. (1989) *The Management of Innovation and Design*. London: Cassell.

Heenan, R. (2009) 'How to beat NHS workplace bullying.' *HSJ* (9 February) Accessed 5/4/10 at www.hsj.co.uk/news/workforce/how-to-beat-nhs-workplace-bullying/1970330.pdf.

Heifetz, M.L. (1993) *Leading Change, Overcoming Chaos*. Berkeley, CA: Ten Speed Press.

Helman, C.G. (1994) *Culture, Health and Illness: An Introduction for Health Professionals*. Oxford: Butterworth.

Hersey, P. and Blanchard, K. (1982) *Management of Organizational Behavior: Utilizing Human Resources*. Englewood Cliffs, NJ: Prentice Hall.

Hillier, S. and Scambler, G. (1997) 'Women as Patients and Providers.' In G. Scambler (ed.) *Sociology as Applied to Medicine*, 4th edn. London: W.B. Saunders.

Hirschhorn, L. and Young, D.R. (1991) 'Dealing with Anxiety of Working: Social Defenses as Coping Strategy.' In M.F.R. Kets de Vries and Associates (eds) *Organizations on the Couch: Clinical Perspectives on Organizational Behavior and Change*. San Francisco, CA: Jossey-Bass.

Hobbs, T. (ed.) (1992) *Experiential Learning: Practical Guidelines*. London: Routledge.

Home Office (2004) *Working Together: Co-operation between Government and Faith Communities*. London: Home Office Faith Communities.

Houle, C.O. (1997) *Governing Boards: Their Nature and Nuture*. San Francisco, CA: Jossey-Bass.

Hume, C., Randle, J. and Stevenson, K. (2006) 'Student Nurses' Experience of Workplace Relationships.' In J. Randle (ed.) *Workplace Bullying in NHS*. Oxford: Radcliffe.

Hunter, D.J. (2002) 'A Tale of Two Tribes: The Tension between Managerial and Professional Values.' In Bill New and Julia Neuberger (eds) *Hidden Assets: Values and Decision-Making in the NHS*. London: King's Fund.

Hutchins, R.M. (ed.) (1952) *Great Books of the Western World, Plato 7*. Chicago, IL: William Benton.

Ibarra, H. and Lineback, K. (2005) 'What's your story? Managing yourself.' *Harvard Business Review 83*, 1, 65–71.

Illich, I. (1990) *Limits to Medicine: Medical Nemesis – The Expropriations of Health*. London: Penguin.

Institute for Safe Medical Practices (ISMP) (2004) 'Intimidation: Practitioners speak up about this unresolved problem (Part1)' Accessed 14/4/11 at https://ismp.org/Newsletters/acutecare/articles/20040311_2.asp.

Ishmael, A. (1999) *Harassment, Bullying and Violence at Work*. London: Industrial Society.

Joint Commission on Accreditation of Healthcare Organizations (JCAHO) (2008) 'Sentinel event alert: Behaviors that undermine a culture of safety.' Accessed 5/4/10 at www.jointcommission.org/assets/1/18/stA_40.pdf.

Jones, A. (1995) 'Huge nonprofit system feels pressure to cut costs, merge or get bigger.' *National Catholic Reporter* (16 June), 12.

Jones, L.J. (1994) *The Social Context of Health and Health Work.* London: Macmillan.

Judt, A. (2010) *Ill Fares the Land.* London: Allen Lane.

Katzenbach, J.R. and Smith, D.K. (1994) *The Wisdom of Teams.* New York: Harper-Business.

Kauffman, C.J. (1995) *Ministry and Meaning: A Religious History of Catholic Health Care in the United States.* Chestnut Ridge, NY: Crossroads Publishing.

Kaye, M. (1996) *Myth-Makers and Story-Tellers.* Sydney: Business and Professional Publishing.

Kearney, R. (2002) *On Stories.* London: Routledge.

Keats, J. (1899) 'Hyperion.' In *The Complete Poetical Works of Keats*, Book 3. Boston, MA: Houghton Mifflin.

Kelly, M. (1993) 'Taming the demons of change.' *Business Ethics: The Magazine of Corporate Responsibility 4.*

Kinchin, D. (1998) *Post-Traumatic Stress Disorder: The Invisible Injury.* London: Success Unlimited.

King's Fund (2010) *A High-Performing NHS? A Review of Progress 1997–2010.* London: King's Fund. Accessed 15/6/12 at www.kingsfund.org.uk/publications/a_highperforming_nh.html.

Kipling, R. (1926) 'We and They.' *Debits and Credits.* London: Macmillan.

Klein, M. (1955) *New Directions in Psychoanalysis.* London: Tavistock.

Klein, M. and Riviere, J. (1964) *Love, Hate and Reparation.* New York: Norton.

Klein, R. (2002) 'A Babel of Voices: Values, Policy-Making and the NHS.' In W. New and J. Neuberger (eds) *Hidden Assets: Values and Decision-Making in the NHS.* London: King's Fund.

Klein, R. (2004) 'The first wave of NHS Foundation Trusts.' *British Medical Journal 328.*

Klein, R. (2006) *The New Politics of the NHS: From Creation to Reinvention*, 5th edn. Abingdon: Radcliffe Publishing.

Kleinman, A. (1980) *Patients and Healers in the Context of Culture: An Exploration of the Borderland between Anthropology, Medicine, and Psychiatry.* Berkeley, CA: University of California Press.

Kleinman, A. (1988) *The Illness Narratives: Suffering, Healing and the Human Condition.* New York: Basic Books.

Knight, J. (1998) 'Models of Health.' In J. Germov (ed.) *Second Opinion: An Introduction to Health Sociology.* Oxford: Oxford University Press.

Kotter, J. and Rathgeber, H. (2006) *Our Iceberg is Melting: Changing and Succeeding under Any Conditions.* London: Macmillan.

Kouzes, J.M. and Posner, B.Z. (1990) *The Leadership Challenge.* San Francisco, CA: Jossey-Bass.

Kreps, G.L. and Kunimoto, E.N. (1994) *Effective Communication in Multicultural Health Care Settings.* Thousand Oaks, CA: Sage Publications.

Kuttner, R. (1996) 'Columbia/HCA and the resurgence of the for-profit hospital business.' *New England Journal of Medicine 335*, 5.

Lakhani, N. (2009) 'NHS is paying millions to gag whistleblowers.' *Independent* (1 November), 1–10. Accessed 4/3/10 at www.independent.co.uk/lions-to-gag-whistleblo.

Langley, M. (1998) 'Nuns' zeal for profits shapes hospital chain, wins Wall Street fans.' *Wall Street Journal* (7 January), 1A.

Lawrence, G. (1989) *Social Dreaming for the Management of Change: A Programme of Dialogues.* London: Grubb Institute.

Lawrence, P. (1964) *Road Belong Cargo: A Study of the Cargo Movement in the Southern Madang District New Guinea.* Manchester: Manchester University Press.

Lazar, I.M. (1985) '*Ma'I Aitu:* Culture-bound illnesses in a Samoan migrant community.' *Oceania 55*, 3.

Leach, E. (1970) *Levi-Strauss.* London: Fontana.

Leadbeater, C. (1997) *The Rise of the Social Entrepreneur.* London: Demos.

Lee, T.H. (2010) 'Turning doctors into leaders.' *Harvard Business Review 88*, 4, 53.

Lee, T.H. and Mongan, J.J. (2009) *Chaos and Organization in Health Care.* Cambridge, MA: Massachusetts Institute of Technology.

Le Grand, J. (2011) 'Cameron's NHS reform is no health revolution.' *Financial Times* (19 January). Accessed 27 June 2011 at www.ft.com.

Lerner, M. (1941) *The Ideas of the Ice Age.* New York: Viking Press.

Lewis, C.S. (1961) *A Grief Observed.* London: Faber & Faber.

Lewis, R., Hunt, P. and Carson, D. (2006) *Social Enterprise and Community-Based Care.* London: King's Fund.

Lindstrom, L. (1996) 'Millennial Movements.' In A. Barnard and J. Spencer (eds) *Encyclopedia of Social and Cultural Anthropology.* London: Routledge.

Locker, D. (1997) 'Social Causes of Diseases.' In G. Scambler (ed.) *Sociology as Applied to Medicine*, 4th edn. London: W.B. Saunders.

Long, D., Lee, B.B. and Braithwaite, J. (2008) 'Attempting Clinical Democracy: Enhancing Multivocality in a Multidisciplinary Clinical Team.' In C.R. Cladas-Coulthard and R. Iedema (eds) *Identity Trouble: Critical Discourse and Contested Identities*. Basingstoke: Palgrave Macmillan.

Lowry, S.P. (1982) *Familiar Mysteries: The Truth in Myth*. New York: Oxford University Press.

Lublin, N. (2010) *Zilch: The Power of Zero in Business*. London: Penguin.

Lupton, D. (1994) *Medicine as Culture: Illness, Disease and the Body in Western Societies*. London: Sage Publications.

Lutz, W. (1987) *Doublespeak*. New York: Harper & Row.

Lyth, I.M. (1988) *Containing Anxiety in Institutions: Selected Essays*. London: Free Association Press.

Lyth, I.M. (1989) *The Dynamics of the Social: Selected Essays*. London: Free Association Books.

Macdonald, J.J. (1992) *Primary Health Care: Medicine in Its Place*. London: Earthscan.

MacIver, R.M. (1955) *The Web of Government*. London: Macmillan.

MacLachlan, M. (1997) *Culture and Health*. Chichester: John Wiley.

MacLeod, D. and Clarke, N. (2009) *Engaging for Success: Enhancing Performance through Employee Engagement*. Kew: Office of Public Sector Information.

Maddison, S., Denniss, R. and Hamilton, C. (2004) *Silencing Dissent: Non-Government Organisations and Australian Democracy*, Discussion Paper no. 65. Sydney: Australian Institute.

Maddock, K. (1974) *The Australian Aborigine: A Portrait of their Society*. Harmondsworth: Penguin.

Madrick, J. (2012) 'Obama and Healthcare: The Straight Story.' *The New York Review 59*, 11, 46 (21 June).

Mair, L. (1969) *Witchcraft*. New York: McGraw Hill.

Majaro, S. (1995) 'Creativity in the Search for Strategy.' In S. Crainer (ed.) *The Financial Times Handbook of Management*. London: Pitman Publishing.

Malcolm, L., Wright, L., Barnett, P. and Hendry, C. (2003) 'Building a successful partnership between management and clinical leadership: Experience from New Zealand.' *British Medical Journal 326* (22 March), 653–654.

Malherbe, A.J. (1993) 'Hospitality.' In B.M. Metzger and M.D. Coogan (eds) *The Oxford Companion to the Bible*. New York: Oxford University Press.

Malina, B.J. and Rohrbaugh, R.L. (1992) *Social-Science Commentary on the Synoptic Gospels*. Minneapolis, MN: Fortress Press.

Mariner, W.K. (1997) 'Business Versus Medical Ethics: Conflicting Standards for Managed Care.' In J.W. Glasser and R.P. Hamel (eds) *Three Realms of Managed Care*. Kansas City, MO: Sheed and Ward.

Marmor, T. (2004) *Fads in Medical Care, Management and Policy*. London: Nuffield Trust.

Marmot Review (2010) *Fair Society, Healthy Lives. Strategic Review of Health Inequalities in England post-2010 – Executive Summary*. Accessed 14/6/12 at www.instituteofhealthequity.org.

Marsden, G.M. (1994) *The Soul of the American Academy: From Protestant Establishment to Established Nonbelief*. New York: Oxford University Press.

Marsden, G.M. and Longfield, B.J. (eds) (1992) *The Secularization of the Academy*. New York: Oxford University Press.

Marshall, C. (2011) '"Go and Do Likewise": The Parable of the Good Samaritan and the Challenge of Public Ethics.' In J. Boston, A. Bradstock and D. Eng (eds) *Ethics and Public Policy: Contemporary Issues*. Wellington, NZ: Victoria University Press.

Massa, M.S. (1999) *Catholics and American Culture*. New York: Crossroad.

Mawson, A. (2008) *The Social Entrepreneur*. London: Atlantic Books.

May, R. (1972) *Power and Innocence*. New York: Norton.

May, R. (1991) *The Cry for Myth*. New York: Delta.

McCormick, R.A. (1995) 'The Catholic hospital today: Mission impossible.' *Origins 25*, 20.

McCormick, R.A. (1998) 'The end of Catholic hospitals.' *America* (4 July), 6.

McDaniel, R.R. (1997) 'Strategic leadership: A view from quantum and chaos theories.' *Health Care Management Review 22*, 1, 21–37.

McFarlan, F.W. (1999) 'Working on nonprofit boards: Don't assume the shoe fits.' *Harvard Business Review 77*, 6.

Meeks, G. (1977) *Disappointing Marriages: A Study of the Gains from Mergers*. Cambridge: Cambridge University Press.

Medew, J. (2011) 'Thousands dying from preventable hospital errors.' Accessed on 14/6/12 at www.the age.com.au/national/thousands-dying-from-preventable-hospital-errors-says professor.

Metge, J. (1976) *The Maoris of New Zealand*. London: Routledge & Kegan Paul.

Miller, A. (1996) 'Merging with for-profits: Flawed strategies.' *Health Progress 77*, 4.

Ministry of Labour (Ireland) (2001) *Report of the Task Force on the Prevention of Workplace Bullying*. Dublin: Government Publications.

Mintzberg, H. (2009) *Managing*. Harlow: Pearson.

Mirvis, P.H. and Marks, M.L. (1992) *Managing the Merger: Making It Work*. Paramus, NJ: Prentice Hall.

Mitford, J. (1963) *The American Way of Death*. New York: Simon & Schuster.

Morey, M.M. and Piderit, J.J. (2005) *Catholic Higher Education: A Culture in Crisis*. Oxford: Oxford University Press.

Morgan, G. (1986) *Images of Organization*. Beverly Hills, CA: Sage Publications.

Morgan, O. (1998) *Who Cares? The Great British Health Debate*. Oxford: Radcliffe Medical Press.

Morley, P. (1978) 'Culture and the Cognitive World of Traditional Medical Beliefs: Some Preliminary Considerations.' In P. Morley and R. Wallis (eds) *Culture and Curing: Anthropological Perspectives on Traditional Medical Beliefs and Practices*. London: Peter Owen.

Morton, A. and Cornwell, J. (2009) 'What's the difference between a hospital and a bottling factory?' *British Medical Journal 339*.

Mosko, M.S. and Damon, F.H. (eds) (2005) *On the Order of Chaos: Social Anthropology and the Science of Chaos*. New York: Berghahn.

Mott, B.J. (1986) 'Whither the soul of health care?' In R.M.F. Southby and W. Greenberg (eds) *The For-Profit Hospital*. Columbus, OH: Battelle Press.

Mountford, J. and Webb, C. (2009) 'When clinicians lead.' *McKinsey Quarterly* (February).

Mudd, J.O. (2009) 'When knowledge and skill aren't enough: Leadership formation takes leaders to new levels.' *Health Progress 90*, 5, 26–32.

Namie, G. and Namie, R. (2000) *The Bully at Work*. Naperville, IL: Sourcebooks.

'Nations and their past.' (1996) *The Economist* (21 December).

Navarro, V. (1994) *The Politics of Health Policy: The US Reforms 1980–1994*. Oxford: Blackwell.

Neale, S. and Neale, G. (2005) 'Clinical leadership in the provision of hospital care.' *British Medical Journal 330* (28 May).

Needham, A.W. (2003) *Workplace Bullying: The Costly Secret*. London: Penguin.

Nelson, L.J. (2009) *Diagnosis Critical: The Urgent Threats Confronting Catholic Health Care*. Huntington, IN: Our Sunday Visitor.

Neuberger, J. (2002) 'The Values Project.' In B. New and J. Neuberger (eds) *Hidden Assets: Values and Decision-Making in the NHS*. London: King's Fund.

Neuhauser, P.C. (1988) *Tribal Warfare in Organizations*. New York: Harper Business.

NHS Confederation (2010) *Lessons from the History of Reorganisation*. London: NHS Confederation.

Noer, D.M. (1993) *Healing the Wounds: Overcoming the Trauma of Layoffs and Revitalizing Downsized Organizations*. San Francisco, CA: Jossey-Bass.

'Non-profits under pressure.' (2001) *The Economist* (27 January), 71.

Norman, J. (2010) *The Big Society: The Anatomy of the New Politics*. Buckingham: University of Buckingham Press.

NSW Government (2009) *Caring Together: The Health Action Plan for NSW*. Sydney: NSW Department of Health.

NSW Independent Panel (2009) *Independent Panel: Caring Together: The Health Action Plan for NSW State 1 Progress Report (October 2009)*. Sydney: NSW Independent Panel.

NSW Independent Panel (2010a) *Independent Panel: Caring Together: The Health Action Plan for NSW: Second Progress Report (June 2010)*. Sydney: NSW Independent Panel.

NSW Independent Panel (2010b) *Independent Panel: Caring Together: The Health Action Plan for NSW – Third Progress Report November 2010*. Sydney: NSW Independent Panel.

NSW Independent Panel (2011) *Final Progress Report on the Implementation of the Government's Response to the Special Commission of Inquiry into Acute Care Services in NSW Hospitals (July 2011)*. Sydney: NSW Independent Panel.

Nussbaum, M.C. (2011) *Not for Profit: Why Democracy Needs the Humanities*. Princeton, NJ: Princeton University Press.

'Obama adjusts a rule covering contraceptives.' (2012) *Times Digest* (11 February,), 1.

'Obama's "war on religion".' (2012) *The Economist* (11 February), 40.

Obholzer, A. (1996) 'Managing Social Anxieties in Public Sector Organizations.' In A. Obholzer and V.Z. Roberts (eds) *The Unconscious at Work: Individual and Organizational Stress in the Human Services*. London: Routledge.

O'Hagen, A. (2011) *London Review of Books* (3 March).

Olson, L.K. (2010) *The Politics of Medicaid*. New York: Columbia University Press.

Oram, M. and Wellins, R.S. (1995) *Re-Engineering's Missing Ingredient: The Human Factor*. London: Institute of Personnel and Development.

O'Sullivan, M.M.K. (1995) *A Cause of Trouble'? Irish Nuns and English Clerics.* Sydney: Crossing Press.

Palmer, G.R. and Ho, M.T. (2008) *Health Economics: A Critical and Global Analysis.* Basingstoke: Palgrave Macmillan.

Papps, E. and Olssen, M. (1997) *Doctoring Childbirth and Regulating Midwifery in New Zealand: A Foucauldian Perspective.* Palmerston North, NZ: Dunmore.

Parkin, P. (2009) *Managing Change in Healthcare: Using Action Research.* London: Sage Publications.

Parsons, T. (1970) *The Social System.* London: Routledge & Kegan Paul.

Pattison, S. (2000) *Shame: Theory, Therapy, Theology.* Cambridge: Cambridge University Press.

Peters, T.J. and Waterman, R.H. (1982) *In Search of Excellence: Lessons from America's Best-Run Companies.* New York: Harper & Row.

Pilch, J.J. and Malina, B.J. (eds) (1993) *Biblical Social Values and their Meaning.* Peabody, MA: Hendrickson.

Pinchot, G. (1985) *Intrapreneuring.* New York: Harper & Row.

Plato *Book 1.* In R.M. Hutchins (ed.) (1952) *Great Books of the Western World, Plato 7.* Chicago, IL: William Benton.

Pointer, D.D. and Ewell, C.M. (1994) *Really Governing: How Health System and Hospital Boards Can Make a Difference.* Albany, NY: Delmar.

Pollock, A.M. (2005) *NHS plc. The Privatisation of Our Health Care.* London: Verso.

Pool, R. and Geissler, W. (2005) *Medical Anthropology.* Maidenhead: Open University Press.

Porterfield, A. (2005) *Healing in the History of Christianity.* Oxford: Oxford University Press.

Porto, G. and Lauve, R. (2006) 'Disruptive behavior: A persistent threat to patient safety.' *Patient Safety and Quality Healthcare.* Accessed 6/8/10 at www.psh.com/julaug06/disruptive.html.

'Profiting from non-profits.' (2010) *The Economist* (17 July), 60.

Quine, L. (1999) 'Workplace bullying in NHS Community Trust: Staff questionnaire survey.' *British Medical Journal 318* (23 January), 228–232.

Ramirez, A.J., Graham, J., Richards, M.A., Cull, A. and Gregory, W.M. (1996) 'Mental health of hospital consultants: The effects of stress and satisfaction at work.' *The Lancet 347* (16 March), 724–728.

Randall, P. (1997) *Adult Bullying: Perpetrators and Victims.* London: Routledge.

Randall, P. (2001) *Bullying in Adulthood: Assessing the Bullies and their Victims.* Hove: Routledge.

Rayack, E. (1978) *Professional Power and American Medicine: The Economics of the American Medical Association.* New York: World Publishing.

Reid, J. (1983) *Sorcerers and Healing Spirits.* Sydney: Australian National University Press.

Relman, A. (2010a) 'Health care: The disquieting truth.' *The New York Review* (30 September), 45.

Relman, A. (2010b) *A Second Opinion: Rescuing America's Health Care.* New York: Public Affairs.

'Retailers and the internet: Clicks and bricks.' (2012) *The Economist* (25 February), 14–15.

Revill, J. (2008) 'NHS bosses "bully one in 12 staff".' *Observer* (27 January). Accessed 15/6/12 at www.guardian.co.uk/society/2008/jan/27/nhs.bullying.

Ricoeur, P. (1980) 'Narrative time.' *Critical Inquiry 7,* 1.

Rigby, K. (2002) *New Perspectives on Bullying.* London: Jessica Kingsley Publishers.

Roberts, S. (1979) *Order and Dispute.* Harmondsworth: Pelican.

Robinson, G. (2007) *The Challenges of Leadership in the NHS.* London: NHS Confederation.

Rodwell, J., Noblet, A., Demir, D. and Steane, P. (2009) 'The impact of the work conditions of allied health professionals on satisfaction, commitment and psychological distress.' *Health Care Management Review 34,* 3, 205–293.

Rowan, M. (2011) 'Amid promise and peril, hold mission high.' *Health Progress 92,* 2.

Rowan, R. (1986) *The Intuitive Manager.* New York: Berkley.

Sacks, O. (1985) *The Man Who Mistook His Wife for a Hat and Other Clinical Tales.* New York: Summit Books.

Salmond, A. (1975) *Hui: A Study of Maori Ceremonial Gatherings.* Wellington NZ: A.H. & A.W. Reed,

Sandel, M. (2009) 'A New Citizenship.' 2009 Reith Lectures. Accessed 13 June 2012 at www.abc.net.au/rn/bigideas/stories/2009/2609699.htm.

Saul, J.R. (1992) *Voltaire's Bastards: The Dictatorship of Reason in the West.* London: Penguin.

Saul, J.R. (1995) *The Unconscious Civilization.* New York: Penguin.

Saunders, C. (1997) 'Hospices Worldwide: A Mission Statement.' In C. Saunders and R. Kastenbaum (eds) *Hospice Care on the International Scene.* New York: Springer.

Saunders, P. (2002) *The Ends and Means of Welfare: Coping with Economic and Social Change in Australia.* Cambridge: Cambridge University Press.

Scambler, G. (1997) 'Deviance, Sick Role and Stigma.' In G. Scambler (ed.) *Sociology as Applied to Medicine,* 4th edn. London: W.B. Saunders.

Schaef, A.W. and Fassel, D. (1990) *The Addictive Organization.* San Francisco, CA: Harper & Row.

Schein, E.H. (1985) *Organizational Culture and Leadership*. San Francisco, CA: Jossey-Bass.
Schein, E.H. (1987) *Organizational Culture and Leadership*. San Francisco, CA: Jossey-Bass.
Schoeck, H. (1966) *Envy: A Theory of Social Behaviour*. Indianapolis, IN: Liberty Press.
Scott, J., Blanshard, C. and Child, S. (2008) 'Workplace bullying of junior doctors: A cross sectional questionnaire survey.' *New Zealand Medical Journal Digest 121*, 1282, 13–15.
Seedhouse, D. (1996) 'Theory or Practice?' In D. Seedhouse (ed.) *Reforming Health Care: The Philosophy and Practice of International Health Reform*. Chichester: John Wiley.
Sexton, J.B., Thomas, E.J. and Helmreich, R.L. (2000) 'Error, stress, and teamwork in medicine and aviation: Cross sectional surveys.' *British Medical Journal 320* (18 March), 745–749.
Sherer, J. (1994) 'Corporate cultures.' *Hospitals and Health Networks* (5 May), 19–22.
Shore, C. and Wright, S. (2000) 'Coercive Accountability.' In Marilyn Strathern (ed.) *Audit Cultures: Anthropological Studies in Accountability, Ethics, and the Academy*. London: Routledge.
Shortell, S.M., Gillies, R., Anderson, D.A., Erickson, K.M. and Mitchell, J.B. (2000) *Remaking Health Care in America: The Evolution of Organized Delivery Systems*. San Francisco, CA: Jossey-Bass.
Simpson, J. (1994) 'Doctors and management – why bother?' *British Medical Journal 309* (3 December).
Smith, P. and Riley, A. (2009) *Cultural Theory: An Introduction*. Oxford: Blackwell.
Smith, R. (1994) 'The rise of Stalinism in the NHS.' *British Medical Journal 309* (17 December).
Smith, R. (2001) 'Why are doctors so unhappy?' *British Medical Journal 322* (5 May), 1073–1074.
Smith, R. (2003) 'What doctors and managers can learn from each other.' *British Medical Journal 326* (22 March).
Spacks, P. (1986) *Gossip*. Chicago, IL: University of Chicago Press.
Spink, K. (2006) *The Miracle, The Message, The Story: Jean Vanier*. London: Darton, Longman and Todd.
Stacey, M. (1988) *The Sociology of Health and Healing*. London: Routledge.
Stacey, R.D. (1993) *The Chaos Frontier: Creative Strategic Control for Business*. Oxford: Butterworth-Heinemann.
Staub, E. (1989) *The Roots of Evil: The Origins of Genocide and Other Group Violence*. Cambridge: Cambridge University Press.
Steinfels, P. (1995) 'Catholic identity: Emerging consensus.' *Origins 25*, 11.
Steinfels, P. (2003) *A People Adrift: The Crisis of the Roman Catholic Church in America*. New York: Simon & Schuster.
Stewart, J. (2009) *Public Policy Values*. Basingstoke: Palgrave Macmillan.
Symington, N. (1994) *Emotion and Spirit*. London: Cassell.
Talone, P.A. (2006) 'CHA mission leaders survey.' *Health Progress 87*, 2.
Taylor, B., Chait, R.P. and Holland, T.P. (1996) 'The new work of the nonprofit board.' *Harvard Business Review 74*, 5.
Taylor, C. (2001) 'Roman Catholic health care identity and mission.' *Christian Bioethics 7*, 1, 29–30, 44–45.
Taylor, C. (2007) *The Secular Age*. Cambridge: Cambridge University Press.
Taylor, S. and Field, D. (1997) *Sociology of Health and Health Care*. Oxford: Blackwell.
Tepperman, L. and Curtis, J. (2011) *Social Problems: A Canadian Perspective*, 3rd edn. Don Mills, Toronto: Oxford University Press.
'The shackled boss.' (2012) *The Economist* (21 January), 68.
Thomas, H. and Pattison, S. (2010) 'Health Care Professions and their Changing Values: Pulling Professions Together.' In S. Pattison, B. Hannigan, R. Pill and H. Thomas (eds) *Emerging Values in Health Care*. London: Jessica Kingsley Publishers.
Thorne, M.L. (1997) 'Myth-management in the NHS.' *Journal of Management in Medicine 11*, 3, 172.
Tolkein, J.R.R. (1968) *The Tolkein Reader*. Princeton, NJ: Princeton University Press.
Trocchio, J. (2011) 'Get outside the tent: Embrace community.' *Health Progress 92*, 2.
Trompf, G.W. (1994) *Payback: The Logic of Retribution in Melanesian Religions*. Cambridge: Cambridge University Press.
Tuckwell, G. (1991) 'Christian health: A ministry to the whole person.' *Catholic Medical Quarterly 42*, 2.
Turner, B.S. (1995) *Medical Power and Social Knowledge*, 2nd edn. London: Sage Publications.
Turner, V. (1967) *The Forest of Symbols: Aspects of Ndembu Rituals*. Ithaca, NY: Cornell University Press.
Turner, V. (1969) *The Ritual Process: Structure and Anti-Structure*. New York: Aldine.
Turner, V. (1974) *Dramas, Fields and Metaphors: Symbolic Action in Human Society*. New York: Cornell University Press.
UNISON (2003) *Bullying at Work*. London: UNISON. Accessed 15/06/12 at www.unison.org.uk/acrobat/13375.pdf.
US Bishops Conference (1993) 'Resolution on health reform.' *Origins 23*, 7, 98–102.

Vanderhaar, G. (1998) *Beyond Violence.* Mystic, CT: Twenty-Third Publications.

Vetter, N. (1995) *The Hospital: From Centre of Excellence to Community Support.* London: Chapman and Hall.

Wall, B.M. (2011) *American Catholic Hospitals: A Century of Changing Markets and Missions.* New Brunswick, NJ: Rutgers University Press.

Wall, S.J. and Wall, S.R. (2000) *The Morning After: Making Corporate Mergers Work after the Deal is Sealed.* Cambridge, MA: Perseus.

Wallerstein, N. (1997) 'Freirian Praxis in Health Education and Community Organizing.' In M. Minkler (ed.) *Community Organizing and Community for Health.* New Brunswick, NJ: Rutgers University Press.

Walshe, K. (2003) 'Foundation hospitals: A new direction for NHS reform?' *Journal of the Royal Society of Medicine 96.*

Ward, C., Bochner, S. and Furnham, A. (2001) *The Psychology of Culture Shock.* Hove: Routledge.

Watcher, R.M. and Pronovost, P.J. (2009) 'Balancing "no blame" with accountability in patient safety.' *New England Journal of Medicine 361,* 14.

Waterman, R.H. (1987) *The Renewal Factor.* New York: Bantam.

Wenneberg, J.E. (2010) *Tracking Medicine: A Researcher's Quest to Understand Health Care.* New York: Oxford University Press.

Wheatley, M.J. (1992) *Leadership and the new science: Learning about organization from an orderly universe.* San Francisco, CA: Benet-Koehler.

Wheatley, M. (1994) *Leadership and the New Science.* San Francisco, CA: Berrett-Koehler.

Wheeler, B. (2011) 'Nick Clegg vows to protect NHS from "profit motive".' BBC News (12 March). Accessed 15/6/12 at www.bbc.co.uk/news/uk-politics-12722836.

'Where lucre is still filthy: Squeamishness about profitmaking is hampering the government's bid to reform the public service.' (2011) *The Economist* (21 May).

White, A.A. (2011) *Seeing Patients: Unconscious Bias in Health Care.* Cambridge, MA: Harvard University Press.

Whitehead, M. (1993) 'Is it Fair? Evaluating the Equity Implications of the NHS Reforms.' In R. Robinson and J. Le Grand (eds) *Evaluating the NHS Reforms.* London: King's Fund.

Wilkinson, R. and Marmot, M. (2003) *Social Determinants of Health: The Solid Facts,* 2nd edn. Geneva: World Health Organization.

Williams, R. (1961) *The Long Revolution.* London: Chatto and Windus.

Williams, R. (1979) *Politics and Letters: Interviews with New Left Review.* London: New Left Books.

Willis, E. (1994) *Illness and Social Relations: Issues in the Sociology of Health Care.* St Leonards: Allen and Unwin.

Wink, W. (1992) *Engaging the Powers: Discernment and Resistance in a World of Domination.* Philadelphia, PA: Fortress.

World Health Organization (WHO) (1988) *Health Promotion Glossary.* Geneva: WHO.

World Health Organization (WHO) (2008) *Closing the Gap in a Generation: Health Equity through Action on the Social Determinants of Health. Final Report of the Commission on Social Determinants of Health.* Geneva: WHO.

Wright, J. (2003) *The Ethics of Economic Rationalism.* Sydney: University of New South Wales Press.

Wright, L., Malcolm, L., Barnett, P. and Hendry, C. (2001) *Clinical Leadership and Clinical Governance: A Review of Developments in New Zealand and Internationally* (August). Accessed on 30/4/11 at hiisc.org. nz/assets/sm/.../CLAN2litreviewfind.pdf?download.

Wuthnow, R., Hunter, J.D., Bergesen, A and Kurzweil, E. (1984) *Cultural Analysis.* London: Routledge & Kegan Paul.

Young, B.H. (1998) *The Parables: Jewish Tradition and Christian Interpretation.* Peabody, MA: Hendrickson.

Yuill, C., Crinson, I. and Duncan, E. (2010) *Key Concepts in Health Studies.* London: Sage Publications.

Zelman, W.A. (1996) *The Changing Health Care Market Place.* San Francisco, CA: Jossey-Bass.

Index